Darker Shades of the VA

R.S. Christoff

Published by R.S. Christoff, 2021.

While every precaution has been taken in the preparation of this book, the publisher assumes no responsibility for errors or omissions, or for damages resulting from the use of the information contained herein.

DARKER SHADES OF THE VA

First edition. November 23, 2021.

ISBN: 979-8201178833

Written by R.S. Christoff.

Table of Contents

This book is dedicated in loving memory of my dad, Christopher, who passed away while on active duty in the Navy. He was an integral part of my decision to join the military as a healthcare professional. His passing cultivated my desire to care for military members as well as Veterans in a healing capacity. In fact, I am releasing this book on what would have been his 75th birthday.

This book is also dedicated to my fellow Veterans in hopes that they receive the care they so desperately need, and are not subjected to the care and treatment received by so many Veterans located around the country, as well as in certain areas of rural America.

Author's
Acknowledgements and
Disclaimer

This book is a work of fiction describing one insider's perspective of actual events and experiences personally observed by the author. The events described have been embellished to an extent (not much has been needed, as many of the stories in themselves are entertaining), in order to format a somewhat comical approach to the *buffoonery* rampant throughout the VA. Names have been changed to maintain the anonymity of the individuals involved.

Throughout the book when referring to most work-related titles (*boss, manager, leader, and specialist*), as well as to indicate sarcasm, the use of italics has been annotated. The author simply used their ***assigned*** title, and in no way suggests that she agreed with those labels insofar as what the titles *do* represent by no means embodies the designation in which they *should*. Additionally, bold italics have been used to indicate emphasis.

First, I'd like to thank the Veterans Affairs Medical Centers, especially one commonly located somewhere in rural America, where I have resided at one time in my life. Had it not been for that specific VA and their *infinite wisdom* (yes that is complete and utter sarcasm), this book would have never come to fruition.

Furthermore, I must thank my friend Karey who, many years ago, introduced me to the term *buffoonery*. That term was slightly portrayed during my time in the Air Force, yet, it turned out to be markedly more abundant during my time in the VA system. Additionally, the designation is extremely appropriate as well its portrayal of the antics observed throughout the entire VA.

Lastly, I want to thank my loving husband for listening to me drone on and on about the contents of this book and my frustration with certain aspects of the writing. He put up with my obsessive typing and writing up ideas at all hours of the day or night and even in the car on trips made to anywhere. I would often ignore his frequent ramblings so that I could make notes to myself that I could type up once we arrived at our destination.

Darker Shades of the VA

President Lincoln's Motto for the VA:

Upon the entrance wall in a VA Medical Center one should be able to find an etching of the VA motto, posted for anyone to see, referring to the care that our country's Military Service Veterans *should* receive. The motto was coined by President Lincoln as a way of reiterating that care. That Motto is as follows:

> "With malice toward none, with charity for all, with firmness in the right as God gives us to see the right, let us strive on to finish the work we are in, to bind up the nation's wounds, *to care for him who shall have borne the battle and for his widow, and his orphan,* to do all which may achieve and cherish a just and lasting peace among ourselves and with all nations."[1]

The words italicized above were President Lincoln's affirmation of the government's obligation to care for those who have been injured in battle, as well as to care for the surviving family members of the soldiers who have perished on the battlefield.

[1] The Origin of the VA Motto. Lincoln's Second Inaugural Address. (2015). Retrieved from, http://www.va.gov/opa/publications/celebrate/vamotto.pdf

Introduction – Why the VA?

Let me introduce myself. My name is Lila Tarankowski. After retiring from the military many years ago, I suggested to my husband that he find a career somewhere in the country that he would be proud of and not come home nightly, bitching and moaning about the job and the people with whom he worked. He ended up finding himself a job in some Podunk town in rural America. A town that neither of us had ever heard of before. My husband then proceeded to inform me that he had followed me from a popular west-coast beach town to a not-so-well-known town on the Gulf Coast, and so now it was his turn to shine and focus on his career. What else could I do but to agree? Hence this story begins...

Before ever starting a new job, the first person one normally encounters is a Human Resources representative (or *specialist* in the case of the VA) who would typically be the *expert* on what the facility requirements were and how they should best be filled. For example, the need may be for a nurse in a certain clinic, and the Human Resources *specialist* **should** be well-versed as to whether an experienced Emergency Room nurse would fit the profile to work in that setting. Unfortunately, with *specialists* at one particular VA, it seemed to only be relevant if a person was related to a particular employee, and not necessarily whether the candidate had any experience in the area.

Eventually a well-qualified candidate may finally have been offered employment and started working (after all the rigmarole of just getting hired), doing their job and doing it well. Then maybe after a few short weeks of working there a co-worker demanded the new employee do their job, also. The new employee, of course, refused, as their job was somewhat demanding, that of learning a new computer charting system as well as how the facility ran, in addition to actually taking care of the patients When the new employee refused their co-worker's plea, that co-worker then queried, "What *is* your job anyway?"

Additionally, with all of the disasters locally and around the world in recent years (whether natural or man-made) many businesses have instilled a disaster (recovery or response) plan. Those plans are meant to either protect their people, care for patients, or help out in the community. The thought would be to have a ***trained*** disaster preparedness coordinator who was well-versed on plans such as those. Now imagine having the supposedly adept organization's disaster preparedness coordinator approach and ask, "What would you do in the event of a disaster?" And leave it at that. No further details offered as to what ***kind*** of disaster, or even ***where*** it may have occurred.

Or, better yet, imagine having a *customer* barreling into a workspace screaming, "I need Oxy!" (Meaning Oxycodone, or Percocet as many people maybe familiar)? Of course, most people would probably only see that in a healthcare setting or possibly a pharmacy. Still, these days who really knows. How about having someone show up in a business asking for help and then proceeding to tell anyone who'll listen that "*You* can't help *me*!" Maybe a nurse has been seen running through a crowded workspace yelling, "Call the cops, he's suicidal!" Perhaps another nurse has even offered to provide a patient's ***stats,*** like one would in a sporting competition. Seemingly not to care that the patient may or may not be oxygenating well, but rather is in respiratory distress, and not understanding that their oxygen ***saturation*** may be a critical detail in that determination. Better yet, imagine finding an elderly Veteran abandoned in the waiting room of a clinic after all the staff have left for the weekend and all the lights have been turned off. These, and many more stories, and ignorant quotes, are those I have personally heard or observed during the time of my employment at just one local area Veterans Healthcare Facility. Please continue reading for a more in-depth look at the absurdities that I have observed throughout the VA.

This book is one of several about my experiences in the various facilities I have worked, while in the military, or afterwards. I do feel the need to preface this, and probably every other book, by stating that I am a sailor at heart. To further explain a little bit more about me, I have tried on numerous occasions throughout my life to curb my **Sailor's Mouth**, however it has been a constant and almost daily challenge/struggle. Those who know me can attest to this little tidbit of information, that sometimes it just seems to *slip out,* as do many of my personal opinions which may not always be regarded as politically correct to those easily offended. One day in the not so distant future, "The Fucking Dictionary" will be released and it may help to decipher some of the verbiage in this as well as previous and subsequent books in this series.

How it all Started

Initially, walking through the doors of the local area Veteran's Affairs medical center one might look from the shiny floors to the wall of water, which can be observed cascading down behind the patients in the waiting room and think, '*Wow, this is a nice place. The Veterans here must really be happy and well taken care of*'. Unfortunately, not only was that statement untrue for a majority of the Veterans who utilized the facility, but the wall of cascading water has since been removed due to a leak in the mode of containment. Even a majority of the smiling faces and pretentious warm greetings of the staff are mostly a façade, as they continually wander the hallways. One might think that the Veterans really have it made, a beautiful building, friendly faces, why not? I am going to burst that balloon wide open, and to say that upon closer examination of the personnel and the facility; that is entirely not the case.

Now don't get me wrong. There are several staff members that were entirely sincere and caring when it came to the Veterans. However, those people were not usually the ones seen ambling the hallways on a frequent basis. Those staff members were the ones that took up the slack for the more overpaid, unproductive employees, discussed previously, including those gossiping about whatever may have been the subject of the day. Another reason certain staff members could be seen regularly carousing the hallways was because many of them either did not have a specific job, or they did not know how to perform the job for which they had been hired. This reverts back to the other staff members (that weren't typically seen) who ended up having to pick up the slack for those less *able*. Or, in the case of quite a few of the employees, it appeared as though they were simply there to collect a paycheck and do as much as they could for themselves and as little as they could for the Veterans, oftentimes working harder to get out of doing their actual job.

Furthermore, those staff members, mentioned previously, appeared to be extremely fluent in passing the buck. This seemed to be a common occurrence for those staff members, so as to not even minimally over-burden themselves, allowing them the ability to leave work on time, or even early, each and every day, regardless of any consequences to the Veterans. For those reading this and thinking this is just one *disgruntled* employee wanting to air her dirty laundry, read on about how some of the Veterans have been treated by employees. Those very same employees who have pledged to care for the Veterans, and have been hired for that exact purpose.

In the following pages I have provided some interesting examples of what I have witnessed, all from personal experience and observation.

Part I
The Staff

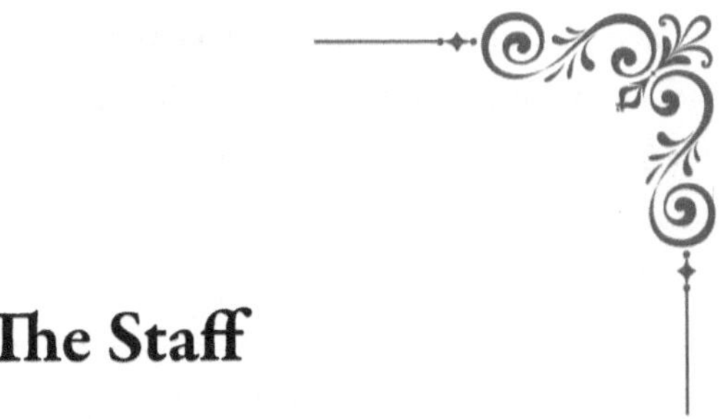

The Staff

*V*eterans Affairs??? In my humble opinion, maybe it should be re-named "Staff Affairs". After all, as I questioned previously, how have some of the staff obtained the positions they had? Certainly not because of qualifications, experience, or knowledge that would normally be required for those positions. Again, this is just my opinion, and possibly several others that have witnessed the same, but most likely not the opinions of the staff in those positions.

The reason I have chosen to call this book "Darker Shades of the VA" is primarily because it is an insider's view of what was observed transpiring in just one Veteran's Affairs Health Care Facility (although, I have heard rumors that several others are quite similar, nonetheless they are just that… rumors). The media's portrayal, if at all accurate, is nothing compared to what has been observed actually occurring throughout a Federal facility such as this.

I had originally planned to name the book "the Stagnant Circus", as what I have observed during my time employed at the VA, was a circus of *oddities* (a.k.a. freak show) that somehow have managed to avert the system and, as of this date, have not caused the entire building to fall down on itself with the Veterans inside. In addition, this *unusual circus* seemed abundant with *clowns* that have somehow, beyond all common sense, evaded reality to the point that *buffoonery* had become a way of life, as the stories in this book will attest. Anyone not able to adapt to the *buffoonery*, such as myself, were found to be in a never-ending circus, as nothing seemed to change. The phenomenon circled round and round like a continuous spectacle, an uncoordinated merry-go-round of sorts, thus a **stagnant circus** — an ever cyclical, yet static circus. I likened it to a hurricane that had made landfall and continued to circle over one area, never advancing.

Flying under the radar for **years** allowed many employees the ability to conceal the fact that they knew nothing about the jobs they were being paid to perform. I say this for those employees that I have personally witnessed either not knowing what all their job entailed, or how to perform their specific job. Furthermore, those very same employees somehow seemed to find a way to expediently elevate the promotional ladder, and still have absolutely no idea how to accomplish the requirements of their original job, let alone their new position. Shockingly, it appeared as though the less someone knew, the faster they rose up that ladder.

The reason they have been able to accomplish this for years, solely in my opinion, is the fact that they must be woven from the very same DNA as an ostrich. Certain people are able to see adversity as a challenge. Others either run as far away and as fast as possible, [or in this case, run and hide, ignore, or evade, (or however it could be described) plain and simple disregard for doing the right thing], or they lay down and essentially *play dead*. A majority of the *higher-ups* I observed at the VA emulated this description to a *T*. Those *unique* people seemed to have actually become experts in doing whatever it took to avoid any type of confrontation, at all costs. From what I was able to discern during my brief employ, the higher-ups would toss their employees *to the wolves* (so to say) if it would save their own asses.

The collective thought processes displayed by those employees, typically in positions of *management*, seemed to be that if they ignored something long enough, it'd just go away, fade into the background, and then that way they wouldn't have to face the problem. This description had been observed in the way those in positions of *management* were seen treating both their staff as well as their customers, the Veterans themselves.

The following chapters describe several distinct staff members, from the lowest level up to those in different tiers of management, and how they best exemplified what I simply categorize as ***stupid***, and it has been well-touted that you cannot fix stupid.

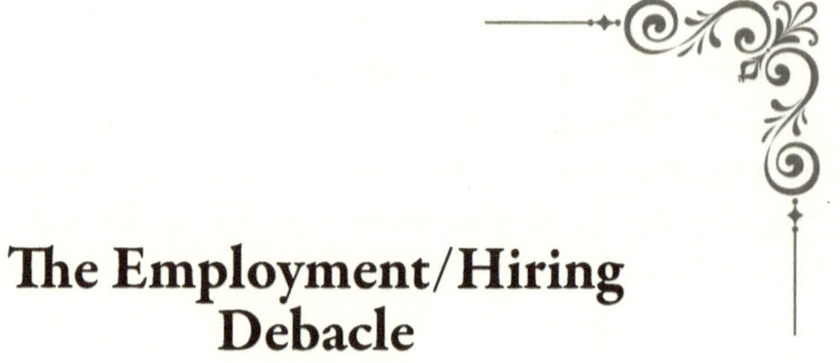

The Employment/Hiring
Debacle

Before delving into the staff I observed at the VA, I feel I need to address the means in which it took me just getting hired on at this facility. As a retired military member, a disabled Veteran, an experienced and knowledgeable RN, with a college degree as well as a certification in Emergency Nursing I felt as though I would become an asset to the local VA healthcare facility and become a strong advocate for my fellow Veterans. I suppose those in positions of power and/or leadership had other ideas. I found out later that many employees at the facility were either kin to someone else who worked there or were *very friendly* with one or more of the employees.

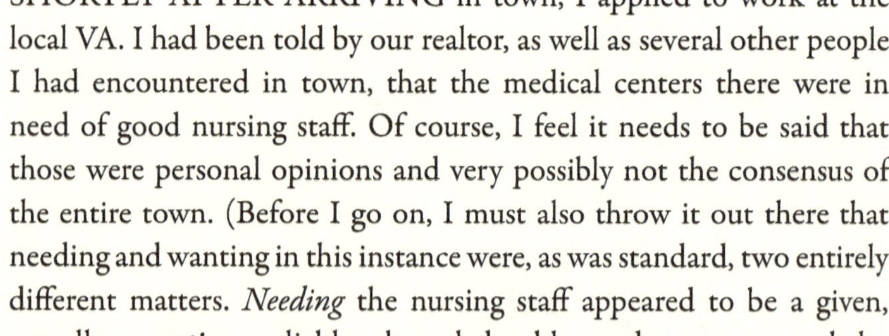

SHORTLY AFTER ARRIVING in town, I applied to work at the local VA. I had been told by our realtor, as well as several other people I had encountered in town, that the medical centers there were in need of good nursing staff. Of course, I feel it needs to be said that those were personal opinions and very possibly not the consensus of the entire town. (Before I go on, I must also throw it out there that needing and wanting in this instance were, as was standard, two entirely different matters. *Needing* the nursing staff appeared to be a given, actually **wanting** reliable, knowledgeable and competent help, however, seemed to be a completely different narrative.). Furthermore, this podunk town in bucolic America, only had a handful, if that, of major employers, the VA being one of them.

Several weeks, (or possibly even a couple of months) after submitting my first application online, I heard nothing. I didn't give it another thought as I was engrossed in cleaning the filthy house and property we bought on several acres on the outskirts of town. After unpacking for what seemed like the umpteenth time in the previous twenty or so years, I applied at the local hospital. I had heard countless rumors and opinions about the hospital, from people in the community, such that one would only go there if they wanted to die, or that was where people would go to die, hence the nickname, *Death Mountain or Scary Mountain*, made me second guess whether I'd ever want to work there, or even be treated there. However, if it was as bad as the rumors I had heard, then they certainly needed some good talent. Notice again the *needing* versus *wanting* help. I ended up working in a couple different departments before I ultimately resigned, for personal reasons, or rather differences in what (I consider) constituted quality patient care.

Afterwards, I did a two-month stint in the local federal prison... that was short-lived. (No, not as an inmate, as a nurse... *sheez*... times were not that bad... yet, thank God.) A short time later, knowing that the need for nurses was still great, I once again submitted my application to work at the VA. That time came shortly after I received my disability rating. Adding together my education, experience in the medical field, a certification in a Critical Care Nursing field, as well as military experience, one would think I'd be a *shoo-in* for a position. Taking into consideration they seemed to be like every other medical facility in this area, short of nurses. *(Right about that time I could possibly be deemed a glutton for punishment. Applying for a federal position is no walk in the park, considering all the hoops that need to be navigated in order just to submit a thoroughly completed application.)*

I received a response via email a few weeks later stating that I was not eligible for the positions for which I had applied. My very first thought was: *Huh?* Followed by, *What the Fuck* (more politely worded: W-T-F – Whiskey Tango Foxtrot; but, at the time I was not thinking so clearly, or politely, and the sailor in me just roared out). How could I now not be eligible for a job that I had done for numerous years? So, instead of trying to call or email back, I drove the brief distance to the facility and showed up on Human Resources' doorway where I was ushered back to a Human Resources *specialist,* Hank who, after I introduced myself, was visually and verbally surprised when he stated "Oh,.. you're *here?*"

Taken aback, I thought to myself, well, U*mmm, yeah duh, I'm standing right here in front of you. I am truly not a figment of your imagination. What the Fuck did he mean by that comment?* Maybe he had assumed since I had an out-of-state phone number that I was also geographically out of state, and that he would just send me an email telling me I was not eligible, and I would let it drop and just go on my merry way. Unfortunately for him, he did not know me, at all! Even a smidgen of common sense would've indicated that yes, in fact I was physically there, standing right in front of him.

As I stood in front of his desk silence ensued. I could not begin to imagine the thoughts that must have been swimming through Hank's paltry brain. I could only envision that maybe when the email was sent, he simply assumed that was the end of my pursuit for a job there, as people often apply to VAs all across the country from their home location. One could argue that there were many Veterans as well as transient workers from all over who had non-local numbers, also. But, I digress. Besides, I in *no* way indicated that Hank was intelligent or blessed with common sense, as it seemed to me to be the contrary. Had he simply looked at my address on the application, he'd have seen it wasn't just in the same state, it was even in *the same freaking town* as the VA!

As my mind seemed to again wander, I noted that Hank appeared to finally recover from what could only be construed as his apparent shock at me physically being in his office. He broke the silence by somewhat kindly, however unintelligently, informing me that my school was not accredited at the time I got my degree. "Well, according to the computer here," he began waving his finger at his computer in front of him, all but ignoring the person standing in front of his desk, "your school was not accredited when you got your degree."

That's a new one, I reflected. Flabbergasted, my response was limited simply to "Excuse me?" Meanwhile, my head spun, as my thoughts are whirled through it and I pondered what he had just said. *Ummm, again, seriously, What the Fuck? Are all these people just extremely stupid or considerably uninformed, or am I just lucky to encounter the only one?*

Once I regained my composure after the shock of thinking that the school I went to for nursing, *many years* prior, and was properly accredited for the military, was somehow **not** appropriate for the Veterans Administration. What?!?!? So, I persisted. "My nursing school was accredited by the NLN. Who does it need to be accredited by, the current administration, because there is *no way* that is going to happen!" Somehow I guess I felt the need to interject a modicum of sarcasm.

Unfortunately, that was probably the first of many signs I would receive during the following several months as a foreshadowing of my time to come while working at the VA. However, after enduring twenty *grueling* years in the military (yeah, that was a bit of sarcasm), I am to some extent, just plain stubborn. (My ethnic and upbringing did not help matters. That just intensified the stubbornness as well as my excessive sarcasm.) In the end, I did put up with the military for twenty plus years, and after seeing thus far what I had in the VA system, at least half of those employees would have never made it through the first few weeks of boot camp, even the *new and improved* boot camps of the last two decades.

BACK TO THE TOPIC AT hand. I had gotten my degree while on active duty, through a commissioning program. By military standards and requirements for their commissioning programs, the school **was required** to be accredited. Hank, in his supposed vast experience as a HR *specialist,* attempted to inform me that my degree had, in fact, not been accredited. :I don't know what to tell you, but that's not on my list here," he informed me, still pointing to the computer on his desk.

Again, I kindly informed Hank that I received my degree while on active duty in the military. *There I went again, thinking that if Hank, in all his infinite wisdom as a Human Resource specialist had just spent maybe five minutes pondering what I told him, he might have come to the conclusion on his own, that the military wasn't going to just let me go anywhere to obtain my degree; the school would've had to have been properly accredited. Who was I kidding? Unfortunately, that would have required Hank to possess, at the **very least,** a baby hamster on the wheel in his head, circling to keep the lights on. That would have allowed him a few short minutes to think about that scenario. He **was** working at the VA medical center after all, with... hmmm,... wait for it,... wait for it... **Veterans** of the armed forces. One might've thought that employees of the VA would be well-versed, or at the very least somewhat versed, in the practices and procedures of the Veterans who had been, at some point in their lives, in the military. How naïve I was back then to think that common sense ruled over inexperience.*

At the time I was in nursing school, (dates are irrelevant 'cause one might be able to figure out how old I really am) there was only one accrediting agency for nurses. Once again, my thoughts strayed (something I tended to do quite often). Furthermore, Hank, the human resource *specialist* as he was labeled, did not appear to be living up to his position title. As he continued staring and pointing at his computer screen he persisted, "well,... your school is not showing up on my list... I've got,..." and he started listing the schools annotated on his computer screen, but all I heard was Wah wah wah wah wah wah... (I envisioned being in an episode of a schoolchildren cartoon.)

Okay, so yes, there I was once again seemingly without a filter from my brain to my mouth as I stated to Hank the *specialist,* "Well, my school was accredited when I graduated, and that was good enough for the Navy. How is that now ***not*** good enough for the VA?"

After I spoke I stood there looking at him, and pondering, *I cannot believe the buffoonery I've observed here thus far.* I then waited for Hank to acknowledge that a little researching on the issue may need to be completed.

And I waited...

... and waited...

... and waited...

(Finally)

"I'll look into this and get back to you as soon as I hear something," he finally muttered.

Once again, I contemplated, albeit my musings seemed to escape in my outside voice as, "Why don't you do that. You'll call me when you figure it out?".

"Um... yeah,...sure," he responded, barely audible.

And with that, I turned and walked out of his office.

TO THIS DAY, IT'S BEEN several years and I am ***still*** waiting for that phone call that I know will never come. Although, I did receive a phone call two days later to set up interviews for the positions I had applied for. Hmmm... if I wasn't eligible for the position I would not have gotten called for an interview. So, duly noted. After that, I no longer made the mistake of believing anyone at the VA when they said they'd do something, anything, like getting back to me, or calling me back. Ladies (and possibly even gentlemen these days), I can only surmise that it may be compared to a one-night-stand that leaves in the morning muttering "I'll call ya." You know you're never gonna hear from them again. (I can only speculate as that's *never* happened to me. Ahahahaha...).

Following that initial encounter., and after barely any thought, as well as not meeting many of the people *behind-the-scenes*, I came to the following conclusion: there were **many** employees throughout the VA system that were in positions they were not able to, or competent enough, to carry out. Unfortunately for the Veterans, those particular employees have been placed in those positions simply for the fact that they either know nothing (those people seem to get promoted *right to the top*) or they know the right *someone.* Rumor has it that there were other ways in which individuals gained employment (or promotion) in the VA system (I will not expound on that and spell out what a co-worker had expressed as a way that a select few employees had gotten a job and/or a promotion. The latter also being rumored as a way in which one very *scandalous nurse* was able to get promoted rather expediently, yet still unable to function as a competent nurse, let alone a *manager*. It was exasperating when a *manager* was required to rate an employee's job performance, yet had no freaking clue or notion of what was required to perform that particular job themselves. How could anyone evaluate another individual on their performance when, as a *supervisor,* they don't even know the basics of what was involved for the job they were rating, or even how to complete their own duties???

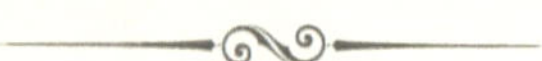

ONCE AGAIN, I DIGRESS. (It seemed to be a habit, I know, I was just hoping that all the incompetence I had encountered, thus far, was a fluke of nature and not the way of life at the VA.)

Meanwhile, as I was leaving HR to run some errands in town, I took the time to quickly look online and check to make sure my school was still accredited. It took no time to assure me that it was in fact still accredited as it had been back when I graduated. Hmmm... That should have been the *second* sign that I was dealing with stupid. I then pondered, how long had Hank actually been considered a *specialist*? Interesting how I was aware that many nurses employed by the VA had far less experience. Many of those nurses only had two-year degrees, and no hands-on patient care experience to speak of. Additionally, it left me speculating as to why this particular VAHCS gave the impression of trying hard to chase away good nurses.

One school of thought might relate to something I had heard several years back. Someone had once mentioned along the way that the civilians in the VA system did not like the *fox guarding the hen-house*. Meaning that they would much rather prefer civilians employed there who did not know how the system worked (or rather *should* have worked) and could be manipulated and in essence kept in the dark, rather than prior military folks who knew how the system *should* run and may force the issue more so than civilians would ever try.

LO AND BEHOLD, A DAY after my visit with Hank, I received a call scheduling interviews the following week for the two jobs that I had initially applied. After the interviews were finished, almost two months passed and I still had heard absolutely ***nothing!*** Including the fact that maybe they had hired someone else on in my place. I again speculated that as short of nurses the VA touted they were (***time and time again***), I would've thought they'd want to hire swiftly, even if that meant hiring someone who was possibly over-qualified for a generic staff nurse position, as myself, or other local nurses. (Maybe that was the problem, I was over-qualified to function as a staff nurse, possibly considering I seemed to know more than most of the managers I had encountered. *HA!*).

Around that same time, two months after my interviews had passed, the VA was hosting a career fair in a neighboring town. The announcement took up the entire front page of one of the local newspapers. I called the number listed in the ad and guess who I got to talk to... *Yes!* The very same HR *specialist, Hank* that so kindly told me previously that I was not eligible for a job there. I decided to play it stupid and began with, "I'm inquiring about this job fair; can you tell me something about it?"

"Do you live in that town?"

"No I live here," I told him, the very same town as the main VA building.

"Oh, well we're hiring for here also."

What did I have to lose? Without thinking I responded, "Apparently not. I applied six months ago and I haven't heard anything about that job since." See, no filter. I have become quite outspoken over the years – from working in a nightclub and a casino, to my time in the military – and I tend to tell people how it was. For some reason, it seems as though people just don't like hearing the truth. I see absolutely no reason for sugar-coating it or beating around the bush. It wasn't as if I was lying, I was being honest. How can that be bad?

Not once did Hank ask me which job I had applied for, his response to my preceding retort was, "Oh, well that job's been filled."

Again I decided I'd play along... "Well, I am a disabled Veteran and I want to know why I was not selected." (Disabled Veterans were *supposed* to be informed as to the reasoning why we were not selected for a Federal position. In addition, Disabled Veterans that are equally qualified for a position as someone else, are *supposed* to be hired over someone else for that position because of their prior service and disability, kind of like giving one a *leg-up* for serving their country. Unfortunately, when the VA could get away with not doing so, they seemed to push the envelope, so to say, and hire their friends and family in the hopes that no one would be the wiser.)

Silence seemed to fill the void in the conversation. So, I spoke up after several uncomfortable minutes of silence, "Hank, any word on this?"

To which he finally replied with, "Um,... um,... let me see what I can find out and I'll get back to you." There was that ambiguous statement again. I knew I would not hear back from Hank. Honestly, I do not even know why they said that, knowing full well that they'd never get back to anyone.

"You do that," I figured I'd just throw out there. Once again, I didn't hold my breath (I might've been admitted to the hospital for an involuntary psychiatric hold, for attempted suicide if I had), and yes, I will probably always be waiting on *that* phone call as well.

Against my better judgement, I decide to show up at the job fair anyway and turn in my paperwork (entire application, resume, etc). I kindly informed the *managers* there that I would continue to check up on the progress. As I had noticed during the brief time of my employ, many people I observed gave the impression that they didn't like performing their jobs unless someone was there looking over their shoulder and holding them accountable. Even then, most of those employees would fulfill their jobs begrudgingly. That was kind of ironic seeing that most military/Veterans I know preferred the autonomy in the performance of their jobs versus a micro-manager constantly looking over their shoulder.

Furthermore, a few times it was so bad that I was able to notice several federal employees would not complete their jobs unless they had a Congressional mandate demanding them to carry it out, and even then, they'd finish the bare minimum to simply get a supervisor off of their backs. I have no idea how some people could work like that. Myself, I like autonomy and do my best work when someone was **not** constantly looking over my shoulder. I tend to get more done that way.

That works for me and a lot of like-minded people. But, I guess other people are afforded more *luxuries* as civilians working for the Federal Government, even to the point of having someone walk them through the steps to completing their job. It has always astonished me what people would do to avoid work. It was almost as though they spend more time trying to avoid doing their job rather than to just completing a simple task.

Nevertheless, I spent the next few weeks calling, emailing and visiting Hank in Human Resources. However, the emails and voicemails I sent must've gotten lost in the twilight zone or something because not one received a response. (Yes, there was that mentality again, trying way too hard to **not** complete a task rather than to just do the job itself, of simple avoidance.) Yes, I know, that should've been my *third*, or possibly **umpteenth**, *sign* that I was in for a frustrating, if not wholly screwed up experience by working at that VA. However, my thoughts were more along the lines that if there were people working in the VA that were that incompetent then they sure needed some intelligent blood to help off-set the senselessness.

So, being semi-retired, I somewhat had the luxury of showing up at odd times to the HR office and checking on the progress of my application. I even went so far as to contact the Chief of HR, Hattie. Wow, she was a piece of work. ***Oh*My*God*!*!*!*** Sooo nothing like a typical Chief or Master Sergeant in the military, or even a competent supervisor for that matter. Not even like any other higher enlisted personnel that were usually in their position for a reason, they demand accountability. When I called this *Chief,* we spoke about my application and I was informed that Hank would pull my file for her to review and she would call me back later that afternoon. A day and a half went by and I did not receive that phone call, either. (Shocking I know. I couldn't believe it myself. Just one more person not doing what they said they would do, how freaking **astonishing!**) Once again, I showed up at Human Resources, (too bad I was not eligible for frequent flyer –

visits – miles), and asked to speak to, Hattie. At my request I was given the blank, deer-in-the-headlights stare by the receptionist. I kindly informed him that I wished to speak to the *Chief, Hattie*. It may seem as though I had nothing else to do in my life after reading through this debacle, but luckily, I only lived a short distance from the VA, and so it wasn't as though I was driving miles to get there.

Once I had the **opportunity** (yes, that was more sarcasm, as it was so not an opportunity I'd care to repeat) to meet with the HR *Chief* I was greeted with a pretentious smile and a more insincere welcome. (I assume Hattie probably thought I was as stupid as she looked because I didn't believe a word that came out of her mouth; but, I did perform the whole *'smile and wave' –pretend to buy into her crap* – just to see how thick the B.S. could really get). We talked for a short time then Hattie walked me down to speak to the Deputy Assistant to the Chief of Outpatient clinics or some other ostentatious title like that made to *sound* important. That person began to inform me of the interview and hiring process, **as if** I had never, ever experienced it, or I was completely uninformed of the process. I kindly informed that person that I was more than well aware of the application and interview procedure as well as the way the hiring process **should** ensue. I then informed them I was aware that disabled Veterans had priority over other applicants that were equally qualified for the same positions. Again, I was enlightened to the fact that the positions I had applied for had been already filled. I suppose that was their *fallback* response. Maybe their thought process was if they told me the positions had been filled then I'd just go away... I told them I wanted to know **why** I was not chosen for either of those positions as (again) I was in fact a disabled Veteran, over 50% with, I could almost guarantee, higher qualifications than the person that had been chosen for each of those positions.

Once more, my inquiries were met with a blank stare and **complete silence**. No answer. I had to look directly at that person to make sure that they were still alive and breathing as they didn't utter so much as a peep. It was almost as if I was speaking a foreign language and they had absolutely no idea how to respond. Maybe I should've tried sign language or even Ebonics?

In any case, once they were able to get a grip on their composure they deferred to a different position opening up in the clinic. (Opening up? Come to find out several weeks later that the position had been *open* for **months** when I was told about it; however, HR was slower than molasses on a cold morning and had basically neglected even posting that position. In fact, there were actually **two** open positions in that clinic, neither of which had been posted.)

After speaking with that *manager/associate something-or-other*, I walked back to HR to speak, once again, with Hattie. By that time, I was even beginning to think that I might've been better off just applying at a local fast-food chain, instead of dealing with all this rigamarole.

Arriving back in the HR department I was greeted by Hattie, who asked, "How'd your talk go with the nurse manager?"

"Well, I found out that the two positions that I had applied for had been filled, no surprise there. However, no one seemed to be able to inform me as to how that happened with my credentials, school and experience as well as the fact that I am a disabled Veteran? Any ideas?" I asked incredulously.

No comment. Complete silence, again. It was almost as if the *chief* didn't even hear a word I said. I seemed to observe a certain trend. One would think I was the *Silencer* or something.

Well, *someone* had to continue the conversation. So, I tried a different angle, "Well, the assistant to the deputy to the associate nurse manager, or whatever their title was, told me that there was a position open or opening up in the clinic. Do you know **anything** about that?"

A light appeared to go on which seemed to bring the *chief* back from la-la-land, or wherever Hattie had momentarily deposited the thinking portion of her brain. She responded with, "Oh, do you have acute care experience?" Being a brunette (probably bottled), Hattie actually pulled off the stereotypical *dumb-blonde* routine to a *T*. That from someone who told me that they would have Hank pull my file and that she would review it **two days prior**.

Really? *Did she seriously just ask me that question? If she had done what she said she would do, she would've known my experience and history. Oh My God, that chief was seriously more stupid than she looked...* Okay, once again, I decided to play along. I was actually beginning to enjoy playing the part of *stupid,* with respects to much of the ensuing *buffoonery.*

"Um,... I *am* a Certified ***Emergency Room*** nurse, does that count?" See, I could play stupid, too I remarked, slowly stressing the ***Emergency Room*** part. However, the operative word there was *play*. I don't think the people I had encountered thus far had been *playing* at being stupid. I think for the most part that was a natural occurrence for most of them.

"Well, we have this position in mental health," was Hattie's response.

Huh? Were we even in the same conversation? That statement was so far from, and not at all related to urgent, acute, or emergent care in any way possible.

"Or we have this position in telephone triage, if you have experience in either of those areas," was her follow-on reply.

It's as though Hattie never even heard me, although I know she did because she questioned me about my qualifications. I truly must've been speaking a foreign language, as neither of those positions had any bearing, whatsoever, on a position in an acute care clinic. Hmmm, so what did happen to the acute care clinic position? Again, although it was wearing me down, I played along with being stupid, "I'd really be more interested in hearing about the clinic position."

No joke, Hattie's response was, "Do you have any experience in triage?"

I think that I might've cocked my head from side to side, sort of like my dogs do when I am speaking to them, as though they were trying to understand what it was I was saying. That's sort-of how I felt, like I was truly not understanding what Hattie was saying or why she were saying it. I really wanted to reply: *Are you fucking kidding me? Do you have any understanding of Human Resources and knowing what experience potential candidates actually have or should have for the positions in which they are applying?* Instead, I played nice. (That started to feel like a twisted sort-of game. For anyone who's ever endured boot camp, that was way worse than the head-games that were played on us there. This had been a head-game where one had to figure out how to interpret stupid, which I found out was **not** an easy task to accomplish... at all!)

Instead, I reiterated, "Well, as a Certified Emergency Room nurse, as well as having worked *in an actual Emergency Room* for the past oh so many years, I'd say yes, I am very well versed in the art of triage."

My mind was reeling by that time. ***Oh My God!*** Wherever did they *find* those people? It was like the blind leading the dumb or possibly the other way around. Oh wait, I heard, through the grapevine, that Hattie, the *chief* of Human Resources used to work at guess where... a very well-known local giant retailer, and had absolutely no experience in the medical field, with respects to hiring. Yep, we had a winner there. Wait... now that I think of it, I might've actually seen Hattie on one of those viral videos, depicting crazy people, that spread like wildfire all over social media. Knowing that I then tried to figure out what she had done (*or maybe who*) to acquire the position she was currently screwing up. It had to be something along those lines as one of the rumored ways in which foolhardy people obtained employment at the VA.

"Oh,... well... we have that job available too. Are you are interested in that position?"

By that time my mind has been completely blown. I seriously felt as though I was in the twilight zone, or some sort of alternate reality. Had Hattie actually been listening to a freaking word I had said, or had I just wasted a couple of hours of my life that I would never get back? What were those people thinking? Right, what was I thinking? They had no freaking clue as to what was going on in their little world, and I was the interloper.

Amidst the chaotic thoughts that were bouncing around in my head, I was somehow able to maintain a calm exterior. I answered her query with, "Yes, that is the one I am interested in. Is it still available?" Yes, I know she just said it was available, but after the conversations I had that day, who knew if it would still be available.

"Let me find out what I need to and I'll get back to you."

What was that, the 'go-to' phrase when someone didn't know an answer, (or more than likely actually not *want* to answer a question)? I was not holding my breath that time either, or even hoping for something to materialize out of thin air from our conversation. I was planning my next step in the whole debacle, even before I left the Human Resources office.

THE MONTHS FOLLOWING the submission of my second set of applications and the ensuing interview fiasco, the searching for an actual open position, and the period in which I was officially hired on at the VA, I chose to do some shipboard nursing on one of the more popular cruise lines. When I returned from one cruise to the other side of the world, I was able to get one of my required certifications updated. In fact, the VA personnel somehow actually managed to get me signed up with one of the local agencies in order to renew that certification, with relatively no issues. I didn't know what to think. I *really* had no idea how that happened with relative ease, especially after everything I had seen thus far. It may very well have been that the other agency had played some part in the organization and scheduling. Anyway, the class was on a Wednesday, and Hank called me almost immediately after class was over and offered me the position in the clinic. After offering me the position, he then asked if I could start the following Monday.

My response, after all that craziness, was "No, you'll have to make it for the following orientation class. That's only two business days away and I have things I need to accomplish prior to starting work." (Considering it had been over six-months from start until that point.) I could've started the day they requested; however, I admit I was being just a bit passively aggressive. I figured they waited *soooo* long to hire me and all the bullshit I dealt with to get an offer, that I would start at *my* convenience, not theirs. Additionally, I wanted something tangible in my hand that spelled out the actual offer, to allay any questions about the job not existing. After all the rigmarole, a hard copy (in writing) was a definite *must have* by that point.

I then went on to ask, "Oh, and by the way, would you send me a hard copy of the offer letter, including my salary?" I was not taking *any* chances, I wanted something in writing in case they somehow reneged on the offer, and I figured it would take them some time to accomplish that.

Then again, not long after I hung up the phone after speaking with Hank, I received a brief, two-line email. I wanted a hard-copy of an actual offer *letter*, even if it was attached to an email. What I got was a two-line email with the position offered and salary quote, *real official*, huh!?!

Well... at least that was *something* that I could prove that they actually were offering me a job. As a prior service member *and* a nurse, if it wasn't documented, it wasn't done, is a good mantra to follow. I was just trying to cover my bases like most normal people would've done in my shoes.

Regrettably, this was just the ***beginning*** of working with *stupid*.

Stupid Does as Stupid Is

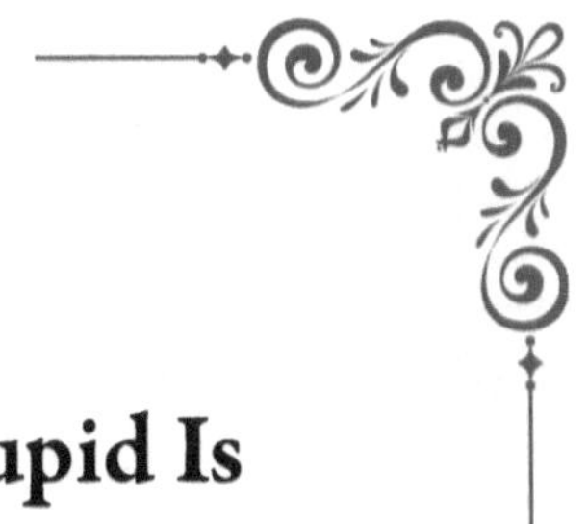

A well-known quote from a movie in the early nineties, wherein the main character was noted in verbalizing numerous times throughout the movie, was *"stupid is as stupid does"*. From personal experience, that statement seemed to ring true for the VA system as a whole, or at the very least the VA at which I was employed for a time. I, however, decided to rephrase it to *"stupid does as stupid is"*, meaning that ineptness flowed through the VA and the more incapable someone was, the more foolish they acted, and the more irrational things they implemented. This could relate to many of the employees; however, it was most abundantly observed in the *higher ranks (or upper echelon)* of that VA. For some reason, the air of incompetence tended to open many doors to the guileless of species. That in and of itself seemed to allow those misguided to perform more inane tasks frequently, on yet a higher level of ineffectiveness, if that was even possible.

Most of the first-hand observed **preposterous acts** came by way of the *management* team. Take for example the realities about Bertha, my supervisor, which will be discussed in further detail in the next chapter. Yes, Bertha was actually **given** the title of *manager or supervisor* (I honestly do not remember her exact title), it was obviously **not** earned based on her lack of skills and experience. The fact was, she was essentially in charge of a somewhat competent group of nurses. Unfortunately, she was not required to display competence in her abilities to perform as a staff nurse on a regular basis. It was no wonder that the local VA had not come crashing down, being led by ineffectual *managers*.

Then there was one clinic *manager* I remember that was as laughable as they looked, hence the *stupid does as stupid is*, they acted stupid because they were. There is a story related to that particular *manager* later on in the book, titled: **Fire in the Hole**. However, they had still been able to pull the wool so far over their superiors, as well as other subordinates' eyes, and anyone else that'd listen. ***All talk and no action*** seemed to ring true quite frequently. It was extremely pitiful that so few people could see what some of the *managers* and *leaders* were really about. Or at least the people that could actually *do* something about all the buffoonery in *leadership ranks*, as many of the employees saw first-hand the craziness that ensued on an almost daily basis.

All the while, those *managers/leaders* continued to tell people that they were more important than they truly were. In my opinion, most of those *managers* were expendable or replaceable. To illustrate further, one certain *manager*, Gus, actually told the local DAV (Disabled American Veterans) representative that they were in charge of *all* the nurses in the building. When I heard that my immediate response was, "No they're not," followed by laughing out loud at the absurdity of that statement. Yep, no filter. I rarely thought about an answer before it left my mouth. But, hey, the truth hurts sometimes. I did feel bad for the DAV rep in that they didn't know, because Gus had elevated his status to make himself appear more important than he truly was.

In the military, if someone were to self-promote, which, in-essence, Gus had done, is punishable under the Uniform Code of Military Justice (UCMJ). However, being a civilian employee working with mostly military Veterans, they were somehow not punished under this (or any) law, it seemed, for that matter. Unfortunately, Gus gave the impression of continually trying to see what all he could get away with saying or doing. And... don't even try to tell me *"but all they need is more 'guidance and education'"*. Sorry, I call bullshit on that! Those employees have worked at the VA for long enough that they knew the ins and outs of how things worked there. They were also well-aware of the *rank* structure and... if they didn't, they shouldn't be in a position of *leadership* pure and simple! But, as I once again digress, that was solely one person's honest opinion.

Most of the following stories are in regard to how many of those *managers* and *leaders* have portrayed themselves during the time of my employment, as seen solely from my personal observations.

Bertha

Shortly after being hired on, I had the chance to speak with my *boss,* Bertha. The title *boss* is used **very** loosely throughout this book, given that I think of a typical boss as someone able to **lead** or **supervise** their subordinates. Bertha unfortunately was unable to perform those simple tasks required of an effective boss. To this day her exact function remains a mystery to me. Bertha's title was, in fact, the nurse *manager/ supervisor* of our department. However, as a nurse *manager* she displayed a comparative lack of ability to perform the basic functions of a competent nurse or even the functions of a new graduate nurse, let alone someone who is a leader.

When introduced to Bertha, I visualized someone performing the role of an experienced *leader or supervisor.* By most accounts that would denote someone who was proficient in *leading* or *supervising* people, as well as someone with the knowledge and experience – or at the very least, familiar with the basic roles of the people they were *leading.* Regrettably, those skills remained unattainable in Bertha's case. The complete lack of being able to carry out the essential functions of the staff Bertha *supervised* was embodied by the simple fact that she was never able to fill in as needed. Such times were those when her subordinates were short-staffed or required additional assistance, usually during busy times.

To make matters worse for the VA and the Veterans that received care there, by the time I left, Bertha was not only in charge of the clinic in which I worked, but a couple of months after I arrived, it was somehow determined by the *powers-that-be* it would be a good plan to pile on yet **another** clinic for Bertha to *manage*. Gus, the *manager* of the other clinic, somehow in the midst of all the clinic *managing roulette* transpiring, was afforded the opportunity of being stripped of his role as manager of that clinic and bowed out of the added responsibility. Apparently he could not seem to handle the burden, (not that Bertha could either). Consequently that task was bestowed upon Bertha to *manage*. **Really????** Bertha couldn't manage the two clinics she had, yet the *higher-ups* decided it would be a good idea to set her up for **more** failure! I guess they (the *powers-that-be*) wanted to make sure when Bertha crashed and burned, that she would go down **hard**! (Oh My God, it really was the blind leading the dumb...)

But, if one ever needed to find Bertha, regarding issues with any of the clinic she *managed*, she was usually in her office, at a meeting (which occurred several times **daily**) or walking around the facility with a cell phone in one hand and a coffee mug in the other. Unless of course it was during her one-to-two-hour lunch break, close to the end of the workday, or on a holiday when **no one** in *management* seemed to be reachable, **especially** for urgent matters.

Yeah, unfortunately, and somewhat frequently, my *inside voice* does not have a filter in which to express my thoughts and, by articulating them out loud I seem to have elicited the dislike by many people simply because I stated the obvious truth. I have often expressed what most people **wanted** to say but were too timid to voice their thoughts out loud. Funny though how those very same people conveyed **shock** when I verbalized what we were **all** thinking. I seemed to have a knack for making it quite known what I thought of how things were run. It was a shame that some people just could not handle the undeniable truth.

ONCE AGAIN I HAVE DIGRESSED. Carrying on (military term for moving forward), during the first two weeks of my employment, I was stuck in orientation classes for three days. Those three days were orchestrated solely by the Human Resources department. Luckily, I had some semblance of a brain, because not one person from my work center, or anyone else's, came by to introduce themselves, or inform any of us where our job site, clinic, or department was actually located. (Some knew, some didn't. I knew where the clinic was located as I had been seen there previously a time or two as a Veteran patient). However, there were a handful of people in orientation who had no idea **who** their boss was, or even **where** they were to report once they completed orientation.

MOVING RIGHT ALONG. Once I started working on the floor I began to question whether or not my *boss* actually worked. Sure, I had met her once, but Bertha never once came to check on us the entire time during the span of those first two weeks, which, in hindsight, would continue throughout the duration of my employ. However, she did come to *visit* us after that time when she had something she needed to pass along, usually bad news, and sometimes a pathetic attempt at reprimanding us (for doing nothing wrong).

Nonetheless, like previously expressed, if I had ever needed to get ahold of Bertha (for frivolous matters) she was usually in her office or reachable by text. However, if we **really** needed to get in touch with her for essential or urgent issues, such as having three cardiac patients (in a five-bed clinic) with two nurses on staff, her response was significantly more sluggish, to the point of absolute avoidance.

I remember calling Bertha one time and, expressing my immediate and pressing needs, as the sole RN on the floor. The gist of my/our conversation consisted of, "We have three cardiac patients here in the clinic, two are being transferred out and we need assistance now!" and I hung up the phone. I didn't have the time to allow her to hem and haw on the phone as I was one of only two nurses, one of which was Leslie, our LVN, in the clinic at that time, and we had patients to take care of. Most other places I have ever worked, that phone call would've been enough to get the boss running to assist, alone if not with a supplement of assistance. Not at that place. Ha!

Unfortunately, as patient care presumably was not on the forefront of *management's* radar, especially *management* that had no clue as to how to perform patient care, it took at least one more phone call in order to get Bertha to actually provide us some assistance. Of course, by that time, we more or less had things well under control (patients were situated – blood drawn, IVs inserted, on monitors and 1st or 2nd dose of medications administered); albeit not the best scenario. By the time we actually did secure some assistance that day it was about **an hour** later, and the patients in the process of being transferred out were either gone or waiting for transport. There was nothing left to do other than wait for the ambulance to transport those patients. Bertha was *prompt*, if nothing else. (Ooops, more sarcasm, pure and simple.)

Deplorably, timing on the previous issue was actually relatively expedient for Bertha, as she often would not get back to us for **hours**, if at all. That was especially evident if we were asking for lunch relief. God forbid she interrupt her daily one-plus-hour lunch to allow us time to sit and eat for ten to fifteen minutes. I truly believe it would have been different if the *managers* actually were fully functioning and capable, practicing nurses. But to have a license and to be able to practice and perform the craft are two entirely different entities in themselves. Hence the subtitle of this book, *those who cannot do lead.*

Onward to bigger and better problems. During the early days of my employ, after finally meeting her, and seeing her significant lacking in her ability to **lead**, I sat down with Bertha, on numerous occasions, hoping to **mentor** her in becoming a better manager and leader. Having 'been there, done that' in the military, as well as several other positions I held previously, I knew how to lead, and what embodied a good leader/manger. However, at that time, after retiring, I really had no desire to perform that function, yet I knew well enough and had the skills in which to function as a good leader, supervisor and mentor.

During the first couple of months those talks developed into a somewhat regular routine. As time went on, it just became more like banging my head against a wall. What's that saying, *Insanity is doing the same thing over and over again and hoping for or expecting different results?* For the duration of those *sit-downs* with Bertha I attempted numerous times to assist in resolving issues in the department, as well as attempting to guide her in ways to become a better supervisor and leader. Hell lotta good it did! It was difficult, if not impossible, trying to assist someone in becoming better at something who did not want or (think they) needed assistance.

It may be possible that I have given the impression that I am full of myself. I am not going to change what anyone thinks, I'd like to think that those who know me, know better and would say the same. However, at this point in my life I know that I have no desire to deal with the politics of the new *kinder, gentler* management or supervisory model exhibited by many companies these days. I personally prefer to work with people who are responsible and accountable in performing the job they were hired on to complete.

I do believe that I've stepped off of my soap box, for now...

HEEDLESS OF MY ADVICE, Bertha continually moaned that she was left in the dark as far as what went on in the clinic. Yes, that very same clinic she was slotted to oversee. Oftentimes she had no idea what was going on, until she was blindsided with the information, and then she attempted to make it **our** problem (and allegedly our fault), not hers. I suppose it could've been because we did not spoon-feed her a step-by-step play of each and every patient as well as all the *goings-on* in the clinic that she was left basically clueless. Alas, she didn't seem to care about remedying her lack of knowledge. Had she just spent more time visiting the clinics she oversaw, she'd have known more of what was occurring. Evidently, it became too much trouble for Bertha to actually do her job and oversee what transpired in the clinics she *managed*, as well as with the people she was hired to *supervise*.

Despite the complete, ***self-explanatory***, log that we kept on a daily basis with abbreviated information on **every** patient (abbreviated patient identification and chief complaint as well as disposition), all Bertha had to do if she had **any** questions about a patient was to look up the information in the patient's chart and read through it. Seems simple enough, right? My suggestion to her one day, after her morning meeting and she was complaining that she was blindsided in the meeting because she did not know what had happened to a couple of patients we had late the evening prior, was along the lines of, "Bertha, all of that information is in the daily log. If you're concerned that you might be missing something for your meeting in the mornings, why not stop by on your way out each day just to visualize what is going on in the clinic, so you'll have an idea what to prepare for and you won't be blindsided in your meeting again." That way, even as she left early almost each and every day, she would see if there were any issues that may be encountered before we had closed for the day. (Or, she could've even offered assistance, as that was usually a busy time in the clinic).

That suggestion appeared to fall on deaf ears, as Bertha's response to my recommendation was a very emphatic, "I know what's going on in the clinic!!!"

While attempting to not laugh uncontrollably out loud at her response, I actually kept my mouth shut tight (for once I more or less had a slight bit of restraint). However, thoughts of, *Apparently not considering you just told me you were blindsided in the morning meeting and haven't a clue as to what happened in your clinic the previous night*, did swirl through my head. Alas, my efforts at molding Bertha into a competent, knowledgeable and productive member of our healthcare team, as well as a *boss and supervisor*, were a **huge** waste of my time and energy. (I've often wondered how much brain damage was caused by all of that banging my head against the wall.)

I had several other suggestions, but Bertha was not open to any suggestions, let alone constructive criticism. In fact, the way she told it, she was a *Super Nurse* and could do no wrong. This came to pass later on in the book, where it is obvious I was correct in my assessment. Somehow though, Bertha was downright unable to even take a simple pulse...

That whole intonation about *those who cannot do, teach*. Ha! That certainly did not apply to many members at the VA in this lil ole area of the country as those that could **not do**, also could **not teach**. For starters, how could anyone teach something that they have absolutely no knowledge or clue of, whatsoever, on how to perform the task themselves? So, maybe someone was not able to actually perform a function, but **knowledge** of a skill or task and how to perform it should allow someone the ability to teach that proficiency to someone else. Not in this case. That would've required knowledge of the most basic of nursing skills. For example, the ability to take simple vital signs. Oftentimes this was done by machine. That simple task only required the nurse, or aide, to be able to choose the appropriately sized blood pressure cuff for the patient. Then came the task of wrapping it around the patient's arm, in the appropriate manner, and pressing the correct button. Occasionally one would need to obtain this vital sign via the manual method. Which, to be fair, **was slightly** more labor intensive and took additional skills to perfect. However, it **was** one of the first basic nursing skill taught; and should have been learned in Nursing 101. It does take a little finesse in which to actually interpret the end result of the vital signs attained. Somehow Bertha must've missed that class, as well as **several** others, throughout her time in nursing school.

NOT ONLY WAS BERTHA seemingly intellectually challenged with regards to obtaining vital signs – specifically blood pressure – (yes, as previously described), she was also unable to tell the difference between a fax machine and a printer. Yes, I realize some look quite a lot alike (**not really**); however, most fax machines I've ever used actually have buttons with numbers on them to dial the number in which one was trying to send a fax. Most simple printers did not have that function, especially at the time this occurred.

This topic came to light when we had our first staff meeting since I had begun working at the VA. Except, the staff meeting was to welcome my friend who had just started working in the clinic with me, and *five months* after I began working there. Bertha sent out an email a day prior to the anticipated staff meeting telling us that the meeting would commence (no, she didn't actually use that word) at a specific time the following morning.

Flash back several months. I received an earful from Bertha one day when she probably thought she might've actually liked me as an employee (Maybe she thought I was a "yes man/woman"). During that time she would often vent to me about her peers as well as *my* peers – her subordinates, (**What the Hell**? Very unprofessional!) Bertha actually stated to me one day, "I cannot believe I have to hire a nurse from outside of the facility." (Instead of hiring her own friends, I supposed.) "There are plenty of other nurses that *want* that job."

Filter-less, I responded with, "But, could those other nurses actually *do* the job in an acute care setting?" Truthful as it was, that comment didn't go over too well with Bertha.

Additionally, there were *two* openings for positions in our clinic, one reason we were chronically short-staffed. And, the VA, or the rural, surrounding, town for that matter, was not overflowing with nursing talent specific to an acute care or emergency clinic setting. But, I suppose if a nurse *manager* with no actual nursing experience could *manage* a clinic or two, then any nurse with a piece of paper (degree) could work in an acute care setting and maybe even be fully qualified for *any* position in the VA Healthcare System. Furthermore, as previously stated, there were two positions open that Human Resources had not even released to the public, or even posted to the job board as available. **Slow*As*Molasses** seemed the way of this VA, as well as many others from what I've been told; however, I have not had the opportunity to experience any other, personally. Also, why was Bertha even telling me that, God only knew. As a *manager*, she should **not** have vented to her subordinates.

BACK TO THE DAY OF the staff meeting. Bertha showed up, a full half hour earlier than she had set the meeting and queried, "Where's Chloe? We've got a staff meeting this morning."

"I believe she went to get some coffee. The meeting is not scheduled for another half an hour," I informed Bertha.

"Oh shucks! I forgot to write down the time." (Yes, that was our *manager*!!! And, she was the one that set up the meeting as well as sent out the email the day before!!!)

"Your email that you sent out **yesterday** (I felt the need to emphasize), stated the meeting is at eight. It's only seven-thirty. It's not for another half an hour." For some reason I felt the burning need to clarify the time. (What the hell? She was the one that set up the meeting as well as set the time.) I pulled up her email and informed her after verifying the time. "I'll print the email out for you if you would like to see it," as I was sitting on one side of the counter at the nurse's station and Bertha was on the other facing me (lucky me).

I found it extremely difficult to maintain a professional composure when faced with such obvious stupidity. In fact, I got in trouble (yelled at and basically threatened) way back in boot camp for rolling my eyes at the statement of someone who was being stupid, as well as not even included in the conversation I was having with my Company

Commander. From someone I was **not even** talking to. At this point in my life and career, though (it has been over twenty years since that time), I have been somewhat able to compose myself and just *smile and wave* so to say.

Apparently trying to cover from her obvious inattention, Bertha stated, "It's no big deal. I just wanted to welcome Chloe during our staff meeting. This is the first one since she arrived."

As usual, I once again responded, without thinking, "This is the first staff meeting since *I* arrived." That just fell out, no filter. **Oh* My * God**, if looks could kill! I caught a look from Bertha as though she'd like to kill me right then and there with her bare hands, and I'd have been dead three times over. All for stating the plain truth. Ahahaha...she'd have to catch me first! Bawhahaha...But... then she'd have to try to do my job and everyone knew that would **never** happen. (Of course I was laughing on the inside because it was true. That it was our very first staff meeting we had since I had started my employ at the VA five months prior.)

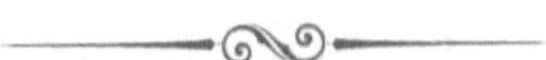

SO, WHILE WAITING FOR Chloe to return, Bertha came behind the nurse's station and performed the whole *shiny object routine*. Meaning, I could've waived a shiny new pen or shouted *squirrel* and probably entertained her for **hours**! One thing I never did try with Bertha was just blurting out *squirrel* when she was around, just to see her reaction. What I am referring to is basically a means of distracting simple-minded individuals by plying them with *shiny objects* or simply stating *squirrel* and watching their reaction as they look around for the squirrel or watch the reflection from the shiny object. That was a simple means to fascinate them, sometimes for *hours*. I'm not advocating for anyone to try this ploy; however, it is pretty amusing. I've often tried a version of this with my dogs by hanging an old CD (For anyone who don't know what a CD is, it's like a DVD. If that does not *compute*, my apologies.) on a string and wave it a few feet in front of their face and watch as it catches the light. It worked for my dogs all the time, as they liked to follow the reflected light around the room. However, they typically preferred the laser pointer.

Again, I find myself rambling.

Making a beeline for the label printer (it was the newest and *shiniest* printer and most, what appeared to be, up to date machine in the clinic, as well as it had the most *bells and whistles* on it), Bertha stopped and stared down at it for several minutes. Then she made the mistake of opening her mouth.

"How does this fax machine work?" she spouted out.

I looked at Leslie questioning as if to say *What the hell is she talking about?*, and then back at Bertha, trying desperately not to laugh out loud. (Oh My God, I could not make this stuff up if I tried.) I then looked back at Leslie and took a deep breath (so that I didn't laugh my ass off and really confuse *poor* Bertha). Whoosah (taking a deep breath and trying to bring in a calm I didn't particularly feel at that moment), I peered back at Bertha, as she intently studied the printer.

I began, "First of all, the fax machine is over there," I informed Bertha, making an exaggerated arm gesture and pointed to the entire other side of the nurse's station, towards the *actual* fax machine, what appeared to be a 1970's model. (You'd think with one that old, she'd have known what it looked like.) Making no comment, Bertha just headed on over to the *actual* fax machine and stared down at **it** for a few seconds (I was guessing because she had absolutely no idea how to work it and, so, possibly knowing she just made an entire ass out of herself in front of her subordinates, she returned to *post* (returned to her original place) back on the opposite side of the nurse's station. Directly across from me once again, (I really needed to rethink my workstation location) to wait for Chloe to return from getting breakfast or coffee.

After a several minutes, Chloe got back from getting herself coffee and breakfast and sat down next to me. She then turned to me questioning and whispered, "I thought the staff meeting didn't start for another fifteen minutes?"

"Yes, it does, however Bertha forgot to write down the time and came down about fifteen minutes ago," I whispered back.

To pass the time, as Chloe ate her breakfast, we begin conversing about who knew what, and old *war stories* from out ER days together, and just overall joking around until our staff meeting was ready to start. (Luckily, at that time of the morning, we were not overly inundated with patients). As our *story-time* continued, we somehow got on the subject of a past patient and the *small* matter of a Bartholin's cyst came up. I was not entirely sure how that topic even came about, however, we were discussing the patient and of course other patients who have had the same, or similar, issues. As if I didn't think Bertha could do it twice in one hour, let alone twice in about twenty-minutes times, remember she's a nurse *manager* - someone who **should've** been more experienced and somewhat more competent than those that she supervised (and if not, would choose to enlighten herself to the topics discussed by her staff without first opening her *pie-hole* – aka mouth – and attempting to discuss things of which she had no knowledge); Bertha once again opened her mouth and fully inserted her own foot when she chimed in "I know Bartholomew's cyst."

Complete silence ensued! Chloe and I exchanged a glance as if to say *Ummm, what do we say to that?* We were both speechless. I then cocked my head to the side, rolled my eyes to no one in particular, and turned back to Bertha, a smile plastered on my face, somehow.

I know I must've looked at her like *What planet are you from?* I glanced back at Chloe and again at Bertha and rolling my eyes for a second time and I thought to myself, *What the Fuck? Did she even know what she was saying? Oh*My*God!!!* I could only imagine what the doctor's look revealed. I had no intention of taking a peek as if I did, I probably would've truly laughed out loud. I realize that not every nurse is familiar with a Bartholin's cyst, however, if one is familiar with it, they know it isn't called a *Bartholomew's cyst.*

When I first started in the ER and heard that terminology (the correct terminology that is), I had to look it up in an actual book, one with paper pages, not on the internet. There wasn't much in the way of internet searches at that time. However, in this day and age, especially as all Bertha seemed to carry around with her all the time was her coffee mug and her cellphone, all she had to do was type the term into a search engine on her phone, under the pretense of receiving an (*important*) email or text, and she'd have known exactly what it was we were talking about. But, referring back in the chapter, I never did credit Bertha with extreme intelligence.

That topic seemed to drop rather quickly.

ANOTHER EXAMPLE OF what I considered PPM (Piss Poor Management), however if you talk to one of the cops we worked with, he kept telling me it was Parts Per Million. WTFE!!!! (Oh, that's the *Valley Girl* terminology for WTF – What the Fuck Ever!) Anyway, I came in one morning, and knowing we had been unusually busy the previous day, I got right to work stocking the rooms and getting them ready for the daily rush. I was scheduled to arrive at eight am, which was also the same time we were scheduled to start see patients, not a very well thought out plan. However, I was not going to arrive any earlier since I was already doing overtime almost each and every day as it was, mainly by working through lunch and oftentimes not getting paid for that extra half hour, as well as staying late. In addition to that, we were scheduled until four-thirty pm and we stopped checking patients in at five pm. So, we then had to stay until the patients were dispositioned (either discharged or transferred out to a surrounding hospital). Hence the overabundance of overtime with being short-staffed and not being allotted breaks.

Thus, I was stocking the rooms to prepare for the day, and Leslie said Bertha called down and was wondering if I was at work that morning. Leslie informed me that Bertha said I was not showing up on the computer as being *online* and *available*. Oh, I had forgotten that the very first thing I apparently was required to accomplish when immediately reporting to work, was to log onto the computer, regardless of whether a patient was in the clinic coding or not. I brought that up because that, in fact had almost happened at least once during my employ at the VA (the patient was brought down from the eye clinic in serious condition from a reaction to the procedure that had been performed on the Veteran). It was apparently imperative to log onto the computer so our *bosses* could see if we arrived for work. That was the alternative to them marching their *fat (or happy) asses* to their respective departments and seeing for themselves if their employees had arrived, and wait, maybe see if they were in need of any assistance. Egad!!! Whatever was I thinking?

So... one of the many days in which we were short-staffed, ... oh wait, I shouldn't say that. Bertha had attempted to *reprimand*, or more like made a half-hearted effort to *scold* me, one day for telling patients that we were short-staffed and that was why the wait was so long. One notable time was the day after Christmas one year. (Well, I wasn't actually scolded that day, as it was deemed a Federal holiday, and no one was at work except myself, our doctor, and Leslie. But, Bertha struggled to scold the following week when she finally decided to show her face back at work, after the holidays.) What happened was that the day after Christmas was deemed a Federal Holiday at the last minute. However, our clinic was required to be open and we were mandated to work. We found out maybe a week before, *after* Bertha had, once again, granted her *golden child* time off for the holidays. (That became a running joke, that the *golden child* would never be around during a holiday because their nose was so far up somewhere that no one should ever want to go.)

Straying the topic once again.

When asked, a week prior to the holiday, what her contingency plan was if we were to get busy that day – being there was only myself, Leslie and Dr. Lynn that would be present to work that day – I was ignored several times by Bertha. I even texted Bertha the day after Christmas informing her that we were slammed. She sent *help* about an hour or so later and then proceeded to try to *reprimand* me the next workday because I had kept the Veterans (our patients) apprised of the situation as to why they were waiting so long to be seen. Apparently, that sentiment was taboo, as I guess it made the *management/leadership* look bad. God forbid we inform people of why they were waiting **hours** to be seen, considering our *boss* was nowhere to be found and made no plans for assistance that day, as it had actually been required. Furthermore, it's wasn't as though the Veterans couldn't tell we were slammed. They saw what was going on and that there were only three of us on shift that day, they're not stupid! In fact, we worked from eight-am that morning until ten-pm that evening, without so much as a break. In hindsight, I could've used a Safe Harbor as a way to get assistance, but I was relatively new to the area and not well-versed in the safety laws of the state.

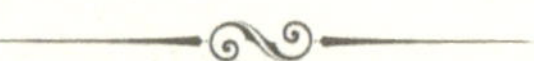

ON YET ANOTHER OCCASION where we were, once again, short-staffed, or maybe I should've said *staff challenged*, we were all extremely busy inserting IV's and drawing blood because the lab was also short on staffing. That was the day that I asked the Nurse Practitioner from the Nursing Home floor if their nurses wanted practice starting IVs (they often called us to come up to the floor and start their IVs as they rarely had the opportunity to perform those tasks). I figured those nurses could possibly spend a couple of hours with us honing their skills for IV insertions, and blood draws. *Oh*My*God*, whatever was I *thinking*? Bertha got wind of that suggestion (a conversation between friends) and came marching down to the clinic the very next day and told me I'd better stop asking questions. *What*??? Wait, let me repeat that... *What*???

She actually approached me and said those words, "You can't go around asking questions."

That comment from her immediately set me off on the offensive-defense. I looked directly at her and stated, "Don't tell me I cannot ask questions."

Flustered, probably that I didn't cower at her *demand*, she sputtered and finally spat out, "I... I... I didn't say that."

"You most certainly did. You stood right there (as I pointed to her) and told me not to ask questions. So, I am telling you, *do not ever* tell me I cannot ask questions." (Maybe I confused her with my reply because I didn't just simply sit there and let her try to lay into me. I was definitely not like that, *especially* when someone told me something so ignorant!)

Continuing to appear perplexed she then spat out, "Th... that's... that's not what I said."

"Actually, it is. You stood right there (again I pointed right at her) and told me I cannot ask questions. I am an adult, and I am going to ask you or anyone else questions if I ever feel the need."

After several minutes and a really uncomfortable stare-down that I was proud to say I most-likely won (well, actually Bertha was staring at Leslie most of the time, I think maybe because I intimidated her), she finally stammered out, "Maybe I phrased it incorrectly."

Ya think? Yes, I said that out loud, in my head... only in my head. I did have a little bit of self-control. But, I did look at Bertha and cocked my head to the side, sizing her up with a scrutinizing glare.

The whole time, Leslie sat next to me having to endure Bertha's piercing, yet shifty eyes (she was never quite able to look any of us directly in the eye), because she seemed to not want to look me in the eye, or even look at me. What the Hell? I kinda felt sorry for Leslie, but in her defense she was trying to chart on the computer and ignore Bertha's stare. After Bertha, outwardly flustered by that whole interaction, (she probably thought she had the upper hand), stormed out of the department, Leslie looked over at me and said "Why was she looking at *me* the whole time? I didn't do anything. What did I do?"

Laughing I stated, "I have no freaking clue. Maybe she's just scared of me? I am kind of scary, don't ya think?" We both had a good laugh that day. That was not the end of Bertha's shenanigans, however, this was the bulk of her displayed incompetence, that I experienced and/or chose to scrutinize.

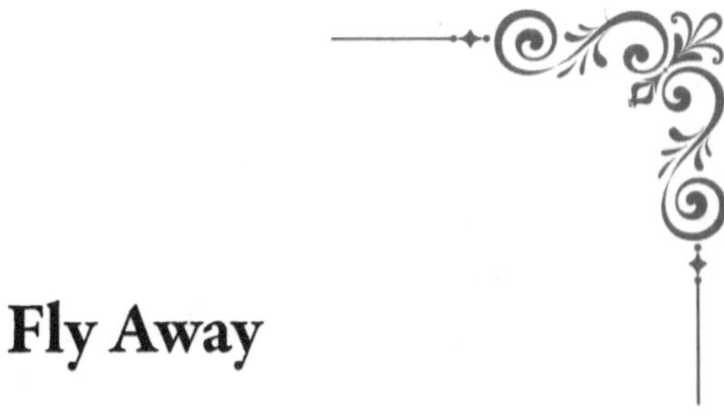

Fly Away

Approximately two months after being hired on at the VA, the clinic was set to execute our first air evacuation since my arrival, (and from what I had understood, one of the few they had since building the updated, and costly, helipad on the property.) Additionally, it was also the first air evacuation for the temporary provider, Dr. Lynn Fitzgerald, who was there for her very first day on the job.

The patient was a LOM (Little Old Man), that I'll call Lou, who displayed practically perfect vital signs, on arrival, for his age, or anyone else's for that matter. To be honest, I cannot even remember what his main complaint had been, which initially brought him into the clinic for evaluation. I believe it was something to the effect of on-going dizziness over several days, or even weeks (I do remember thinking that his Primary Care Provider should have addressed the issue previously so it was an on-going issue), but, as many of us already knew, the VA was typically not known for *actually taking care of* their patients.

To VA providers it seemed like the best-known defense for most patient complaints was just to throw a drug at it and hope that would pacify the patient enough so that they didn't return for the same complaint in the future. (Repeat visits for the same complaints makes the VA, as a whole, look bad, as well as the providers). If a drug couldn't be tossed at a complaint, then most providers predictably did not want to investigate further in order to determine the cause of a patient's ailment, but rather hurl another drug their way and hope that may work to alleviate the symptoms. Although some providers would actually explore the problem and consider other options in which to provide relief, but, unfortunately those providers were few and far between. Complacency such as this seemed to trigger the Veterans to head to our clinic for treatment. That was usually at the point when their symptoms became so bad they didn't want to or couldn't deal with them anymore. Other Veteran avoided evaluation and treatment all together, opting to self-medicate instead.

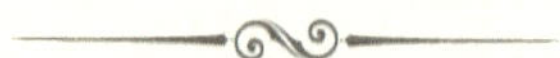

GETTING BACK TO LOU, after having labs drawn and about an hour or so after his first set of vital signs had been taken, Lou started complaining of just overall not feeling well and having an episode of some slight dizziness. I went ahead and checked his vital signs, as it had been about an hour since they had been checked last and since he was feeling worse than when he came into the clinic. Oddly enough, by that time, his blood pressure was in the toilet, reading something to the effect of 70's over 30's. Weirdly enough, he was still awake, talking to us, but he did look a tad bit grayish. (That's not usually a good sign as a patient and not intentionally wanting to look that color.) I must've rechecked his blood pressure about two more times, on both arms, just to confirm the reading, receiving very similar results.

After notifying Dr. Fitzgerald, who had taken over for the VA doctor that was on shift earlier in the day, and apparently had to leave early because, God forbid, she were to work overtime, Dr. Lynn reviewed the lab results and rattled off about five different diagnoses before she even turned the page. Again, this was her *very first day* at the clinic and was getting settled in and verifying her credentials and other appropriate paperwork in order to start the following Monday. Next thing we knew, she stated, "He needs to leave here now!" Meaning, he needed to be transferred to an actual hospital, considering we were just a clinic and did not have inpatient capabilities (or the competent staff to actually take care of a patient overnight, save for a select few RNs and LVNs). Dr. Fitzgerald's very first suggestion was to fly Lou out, as he needed to be in a hospital over an hour away, and the local hospital also did not have the capabilities to care for him, let alone keep him alive. Likewise, his cardiologist was an hour away.

As happened with most of the transfers that occurred after hours, or nearer to the end of the workday or work week, the clerk usually ended up calling around for transportation, either ground or air, (as the VA transportation department regularly seemed unable to be located around that time of the day) in order to transfer the patient once he was accepted at a specific hospital. Unless it was a true emergency, as was in this case.

Unfortunately, in Lou's case, the transfer turned into a complete Charlie Foxtrot (also known as a Cluster Fuck – or rather complete chaos!). Having two new people on staff (myself as well as Dr. Lynn) and two or three other staff members, one being Bertha our *boss*, who acted as though she wouldn't know where to point the hose at a burning fire, made things a little more challenging. Knowing *where* we needed to send Lou, and knowing *how* he needed to get there, as competent medical staff, we did what most prudent people in our situation would have done, had the clerk call the local air ambulance company.

The local air ambulance company was usually relatively quick to respond. Unfortunately for some reason unknown at the time, at least twenty minutes had passed and we all had begun wondering what had held up the helicopter from landing. We heard the helicopter circling overhead for several minutes, but they never landed. The clerk was asked what had happened, but even he had no idea. Upon further investigation, they found out that person in charge of transportation was still in their office and had taken it upon themselves to cancel the helicopter without telling anyone, especially the patient's healthcare providers. This from someone without any kind of medical training or knowledge whatsoever, as well as someone who did not even know the patient or what was going on in the clinic at that time. What's more, it was someone who did not seem to know what was going on in general. So, without talking with any of the providers caring for Lou, nor obtaining any details whatsoever, including checking on the status of our patient, this unseen entity just took it upon themselves and canceled the helicopter. Furthermore, they didn't inform *anyone* of their decision to cancel the transportation.

Meanwhile, checking back in with Lou, he remained stable, his blood pressure, although sadly low, remained steady, albeit at that same low reading, regardless of pumping fluid into him in attempts to improve the numbers. By that point in time, we had done all that was in our arsenal of medical capabilities to do for Lou, including medications and additional fluids, however nothing seemed to be working.

While monitoring his blood pressure at regular intervals, approximately every fifteen minutes or so, from there on out, (once it was indicated), as well as talking with him and monitoring his level of consciousness, he continued to remain alert and oriented and in relatively good spirits. Granted, he did complain of extreme lightheaded and dizziness, (go figure), nevertheless he was more comfortable sitting up in the wheelchair rather than being forced to lie down on the gurney. At his age, who was I to argue with patient comfort? We offered, he refused. As any prudent and competent nurse knows, when a patient is unstable, albeit alert and oriented, you make that patient as comfortable as possible in order to decrease any additional stress that may be placed on them, such as forcing them in positions that are highly uncomfortable. Still, as I had, and will continue to state numerous times, there was **not** a plethora of competent, prudent nurses in positions of leadership at that particular facility, and thus an unwritten mantra of such was, *do as I say, not what is right for the patient,* it was expected that we follow their inappropriate orders. I chose not to, in favor of caring for my patient in the best way appropriate for his comfort. Unfortunately, that attitude was not received well by *management*.

As I continued monitoring my patient, either at the bedside or from behind the nurse's station and well within eyesight at all times, (I mean, five beds in the clinic and all were visible from the workstation), I proceeded to compile the mound of paperwork required for transfer. That all-in addition to calling report to the receiving hospital and watching out for the helicopter, (luckily Lou was our only, and last patient of the day). Reiterating, the clinic was only a ***five-bed*** facility and with the nurse's station in the center, I was able to monitor Lou from my position at the nurse's station, or during one of my many trips between the nurse's station and the door leading out of the clinic as I kept an eye out for the helicopter. In other words, I was multitasking in order to facilitate and expedite Lou's transfer. After all, what did Emergency Nurses do best? Multitask!

Interestingly enough, three or four (or possibly more) staff members still remained milling about, in and around the clinic, some also mirrored my moves of checking on the status of the helicopter while I was at the nurse's station organizing Lou's transfer items. Those three or four staff members, all levels of nurses and a doctor or two, remained in the clinic until our last patient was dispositioned, that was not typically the norm, but that was not a ordinary day either.

During that entire incident, there was always at least one (if not more) staff members inside the clinic at any one time. Additionally, there were lots of other staff members floating around outside of our clinic, for a lack of better word – rubbernecking – trying to view the helicopter landing, which, again, was not a common occurrence, apparently. Included in the sea of *rubberneckers* was the interim *Chief Nurse,* who looked as though she was holding up the wall of the clinic, standing ***directly opposite*** from Lou's room. (It may be necessary to reread those words in the previous sentence.) The person holding up the wall was the interim *Chief **nurse**,* who was in fact a ***nurse*** (possibly in title only based on what I had seen and the fallout from her observations during everything that had happened).

Unfortunately, from my perspective, it seemed apparent that she was just as *competent* as other nurses in positions of *leadership* in the facility, that of having absolutely no clue how to perform the function of a nurse and actually care for a patient, let alone one who was critically ill. If I had to guess, the *Chief Nurse's* main concern was that the wall might fall down if she were to step away from it, and seemingly wanted to make sure that did not happen. (The wall falling down evidently being much more important than the Veteran making it out of the clinic alive.)

To reiterate, the *Chief Nurse* was in fact standing directly across from Lou's room, not down the hall or around the corner or anywhere else during this timeframe, watching him for at least a good twenty minutes, that I personally observed. Or, maybe I was wrong altogether, and she was snoozing on the job with their eyes open, like we were able to do back in boot camp. Who really knew, considering what she did the next day after this incident occurred. (This point is relevant in the next chapter.) Again, she was *allegedly* a **nurse**, that's the important point. (Oh wait, what was I thinking? So was my *boss*, and Bertha couldn't even function as a graduate nurse.) After the helicopter finally landed (no thanks to the head person in transportation, or the Interim *Chief Nurse* who could very well have assisted in facilitating the logistics of patient transportation), we were able to get Lou packaged up rather expediently and on the helicopter, and in the competent hands of the air ambulance personnel. He was finally on his way to a higher level of care. The unfortunate part was the wasting of valuable time in the interim. We thanked our local air ambulance personnel for their assistance.

LATER THAT EVENING we received word that Lou had in fact made it to the receiving facility without too much drama, and only a few *hiccups* along the way.

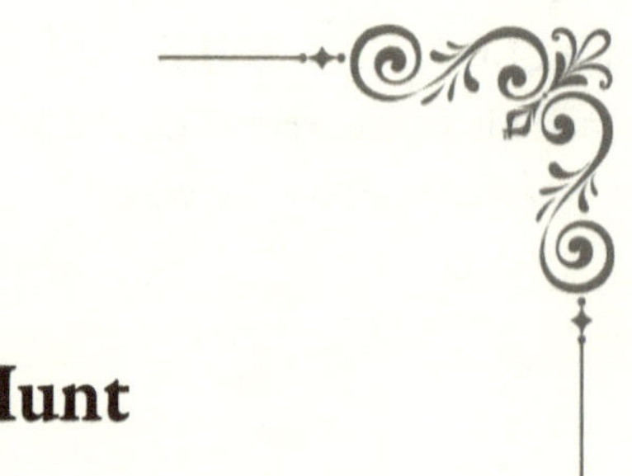

Witch Hunt

Referring to the patient from the previous chapter, Lou, the important point is that he got transferred appropriately in the end and most of our staff was glad that he made it safely to the hospital with only a few minor hiccups, no thanks to the chief nurse at the time. Fortunately, Lou's status enroute and arrival to the hospital safely was reported back to us via the air ambulance personnel. Unfortunately, that was not good enough for the Quality *Management* staff. Bearing in mind, at least one of the staff members in that department was supposed to be a nurse, and I was informed that one of those nurses had been licensed for a very long time; alas, from what I had been told though, the most they have done related to direct patient care was a year at best. Sadly, I did not know this for a fact, nonetheless based on the report they initiated, they did not know **anything** about patient care, let alone the care of acute or critical ill patients. That was the person that *reported **my*** performance as the primary nurse caring for Lou, during a *peer review*. The nurse claimed I failed to care for my patient, sight unseen (that nurse never once set foot in the clinic).

Again, sight-unseen, the basis of their claim was that I was not properly monitoring Lou and he was left alone for long periods of time. The *nurse* even went so far as to state this fact was observed by the Interim *Chief Nurse* herself and the Veteran was left alone for a good portion of twenty minutes. One of their allegations was that I had not documented certain procedures in the electronic medical record, mainly vital signs. I had of course, but they were most likely not in the appropriate place in the record, as I had not received an appropriate orientation on the medical record and I was basically flying by the seat of my pants and fumbling through the EMR. So, the information was in there, probably just not in the correct location.

After my initial shock and surprise that this farce was even addressed as an issue, I began to critique each and every one of their accusations annotated on the peer review. To begin with, their allegations were entirely incorrect. I saw it for what it was, nothing more than a *witch hunt*, as I was never away from Lou for longer than a minute or two at most.

Secondly, the fact that the interim Chief *nurse* purportedly observed the Veteran not being monitored proves that they in fact were right there monitoring and watching Lou, and evidently studying their watch the entire time. **Egad!** They were in fact a *nurse*, which was their primary job, and if they couldn't function as a regular nurse, then maybe they needed to step down from their position in *management* and re-learn their primary role. As a *nurse*, if they were concerned with the patient's safety and the fact that the other people in the clinic apparently could not handle his care, then they should have stepped in and done the job they were (or rather should've been) licensed to perform! Must I go on??? **Oh*My*God,**

I could not believe that they even had the audacity to bring that up as a pathetic attempt at a reprimand. The whole incident was nothing more than a far-reaching witch hunt. Being completely in the right, I wrote a two-to-three-page rebuttal to their *peer review.* I even included specific citations from Emergency Nursing references and standard Nursing journals, spelling out the best way in which to care for patients. In the end, all that transpired gave the impression of a pathetic attempt of getting me fired.

To clarify, a *peer review* is used to review when an error has been made, and ultimately supposed to be conducted by a panel of *peers*, hence the name. My peers would've consisted of those nurses with about the same amount of education, experience, and schooling, which included over a dozen years of nursing experience and at least that amount of Emergency Nursing knowledge. What I was able to gather from people I had worked with and have talked to at the VA, there were very few nurses there, including at any of the outlying clinics, that could be considered my *peer*, to the extent of having significant ER experience or even direct patient care experience.

When questioned about the qualifications of the personnel on my *peer review* panel (after submitting my rebuttal to their ridiculousness) I was swiftly brushed off and basically ignored. Interestingly enough, within a day or two I was told that the decision had been made and the review was complete. And that was that! I didn't hear another word afterwards. I can only assume that it was as though after reading my rebuttal, the entire *case/review* was dropped.

Based on what I've previously experienced, as well as my understanding of the one *nurse* in quality management, they would, in no way even be considered a *peer* of mine, except for *maybe* having their license for the same amount of time. Hmmm interesting! That was just another one of this VA's ways of sticking their heads in the sand and ignoring what really mattered (doing the most to afford our Veterans the best care possible). Additionally, that was a way for the VA to avoid the standard obligation of doing things by the book (also known as the *standard operating procedure* book). I am sure they probably had their **own** book in which they had their **own** set of standards required to accomplish the tasks they needed to complete. Considering the occurrences I'd seen thus far, there must've been another book that only certain individual employees were privy to. **Or** they simply made up the rules as they went along and hoped no one was the wiser.

The employees at any and all Veterans Affairs clinics/medical facilities/hospitals work for the government, *with* Veterans of the military. This should not be a surprise to anyone, considering that is what the VA was for – Veteran's Affairs. Nonetheless, a majority of civilian employees seemed to have no clue when it came to Standard Operating Procedures (SOPs) or Operating Instructions (OIs). All that entailed was following directions; going *by the book* and following rules, regulations, and procedures as to how such operations are to be carried out. Nurses also have a form of Standard Operating Procedures, it's called the Nurse Practice Act and Standards of Nursing Care. However, I've wondered many times if the nurses at the VA were ever expected to follow those rules. More times than I could count I have observed *leadership* at the VA doing what they wanted, how they wanted, regardless of how things were supposed to run. There seemed to be no actual rhyme or reason for how most processes were performed.

In the aftermath of the whole incident, and my scholarly write-up on the proper way in which to care for a patient in an acute situation, I constructed (what I believed was) a well-thought-out and easy to understand orientation guide on how to navigate the Electronic Medical Record (EMR) that the VA utilized. Surprisingly enough, I was not deterred or discouraged by the whole incident and still wanted to make that a better place for new employees, in addition to my fellow Veterans. I hoped my initiative might have been an educational enlightenment for several staff members.

Like any Electronic Medical Record, the specific one the VA used could be confusing, even for those who have used it for years. However, as medical personnel, we tend to find ways to navigate it, even if it means that specific notes were not documented under the correct tab. Therefore, those that have used it for years only seemed to know how to navigate it the way in which they were taught, or learned independently, and therefore have been doing for *years*. The mantra that *this is the way we've always done it*, seemed to be a trend, not that it was in any way correct. Additionally, those that have muddled through the system for years indicated that they were completely incapable of thinking outside the box. As neither I (nor anyone that started at the

VA at the same as myself) ever received *any* orientation on navigating through the EMR I *fumbled* my way through the electronic chart and proceeded with documenting the way I've always done... thoroughly!

However, the way in which I documented Lou's vital signs (as well as many others afterwards) was in a narrative note. That way I was sure that anything I was to do for a patient was documented as thoroughly as I would've liked. And, the fact that I didn't find the vital signs documentation location until several weeks into my employ, which happened to be after this incident. For the most part, EMRs were point and click, checkboxes, or drop-downs and many do not allow for any supplementary descriptive or narrative documenting or any (what some might deem) *extraneous* information. I've always followed the old adage, *if it wasn't documented it wasn't done*, and therefore I like to document **everything** I've done for a patient.

Writing up the orientation guide, I went through the entire Electronic Medical Record, annotating which forms/tabs we, in the clinic, would most commonly need to use. I then wrote a step-by-step guide on how to go about documenting treatments and such. That was my personal way to solve any future issues, alleged or real, for future staff coming to work at the clinic. Unfortunately, Bertha, did not see that as a positive improvement to a broken process. In my opinion, it had indeed improved a failed process, even if it was just at the one clinic. Alas, it made our *manager* look inept in the process. Still, Bertha's main focus was on the fact that I had written in my rebuttal that I *fumbled* my way through learning to document on the EMR. *Ummm, well, I did.* I had no idea how else to describe it. So, so very sorry if the truth hurt. Not really! (I guess honesty wasn't necessarily the best policy.) In addition, if someone doesn't want to know the truth, then in my opinion, those people should not be any kind of leadership position. Bertha's response after reading my rebuttal was, "You might want to change the wording on this, as the word *fumbled* makes us look bad."

Duh! Makes *us* look bad, or just her?

...And...*What's your point?* I thought to myself. It was the truth. To appease her, I rewrote that section utilizing the word *muddled* instead. Sad how she was never the wiser. (*Fumbled* made her look bad, but *muddled* was perfectly fine. Go figure.) In fact, I do believe I possibly switched the wording back to *fumbled* just prior to submitting my final rebuttal. Ooops!

I knew that the entire *investigation/review/witch-hunt* was bogus when after turning in my rebuttal I did not hear one peep from the *Quality Management* weenies. That was most likely because they knew they were wrong in initiating the whole investigation in the first place. To their credit, maybe they actually learned a thing or two about patient care from my write-up, one could only hope. One issue averted.

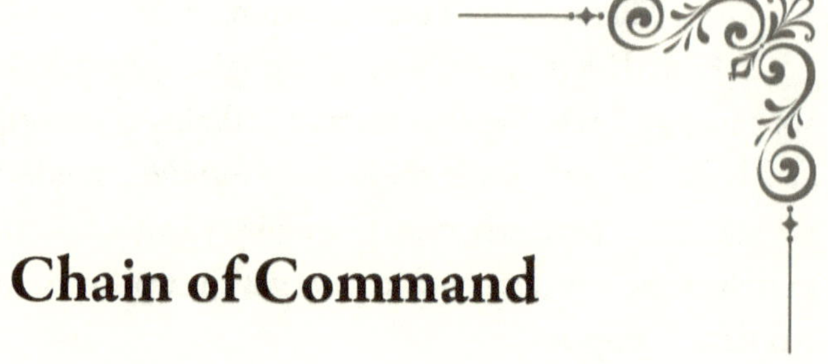

Chain of Command

Now there's a phrase that typically only military-minded individuals can truly understand and appreciate. Case in point, there had been a patient in the clinic with a mental health complaint (we had several over the time of my employ). It was at the end of the day (I think that may have been the only time those patients ever presented to the clinic. I surmised that as probably because they spent the day sleeping and wanted to get in to see a provider just prior to the clinic closing. The alternate thought was that they spent the day in the mental health clinic, obtaining no assistance and thus presented to our clinic hoping for some quality support/treatment). This was also right around the time there was a big hoopla about the VA, as a whole, not taking care of their mental health patients. That was definitely an issue here at this VA clinic. The mental health clinic not only seemed to **not** take care of their *own* patients already registered in their clinic, they would literally pick-and-choose whether they would take on any new patients. After the following incident, I began informing Veterans that if they had an urgent or emergent mental health issue, that their best bet was to go on to the nearest ER as the mental health providers at our VA really didn't want to see them. No apologies. I'm just the messenger and those have been my observations.

BACK TO THE STORY. It was late in the afternoon one Friday and we were in need of a mental health provider to come and evaluate a

Veteran and see if they could be discharged or if they would need more intensive inpatient psychiatric treatment. In fact, it had actually been just around closing time for most other clinics, although *not* quite time to close up shop. I called the front desk of the mental health clinic and spoke with a clerk. Other than our clinic, when someone called another clinic in the facility they would speak to a clerk. In our clinic, there was not a clerk to answer phones and the caller would always end up talking to a nurse or another provider.

I digress once again. I explained the situation to the clerk and requested a provider to come to our clinic and evaluate the patient. "Hi, this is Lila, down in the acute care clinic, we need a mental health provider to evaluate one of our patient."

"All of the providers are gone for the day," was the response I got.

*Uh, it's not even closing time and **all** the providers are **gone?*** I thought to myself.

Not to be discouraged I asked, "Okay, who's on call?" Naturally, I wrongly assumed that I was in an appropriate medical facility that had conscientious providers who *actually wanted* to take care of their patients. Who was I fooling?

"They don't pull call."

"Excuse me? We have a patient here in the clinic that needs to be evaluated by a mental health provider and you're telling me that 1.there's no one still in the clinic to see a patient because they all left early for the day; and 2. there is no one on call that will come in to evaluate this Veteran?" I asked stupefied.

"That's correct," was her response, seemingly not even one bit concerned about the Veteran.

"Would you please send me a copy of your instruction specifying this information?"

"You'll have to go through your chain of command for that."

Seriously?!?!? You've got to be fucking kidding me. Sometimes I thought those people spouted out words having no idea of their meaning. The clerk wanted me to go through my chain of command to get a freaking instruction! That was like telling a nurse in another clinic, *Sorry, you'll have to go through your chain of command to get a copy of the instruction you are looking for on how to properly insert an intravenous line (IV).* Ignorance, plain and simple! That was the only way I could even **begin** to explain their thought process. Simply put, instructions were (supposed to be) available for anyone to peruse. They are not secrets (or rather shouldn't be). They are a means of standardizing patient care.

Knowing I wouldn't get very far in that conversation, I didn't even try pushing the issue. I just hung up on her. By that time in my employ, I was at the point of picking my battles, and short of walking up to the third or fourth floor (taking time out from patient care) to give that clerk a verbal *dressing-down* (similar to a reprimand), I just opted for patient care first and initiating an incident report write up second. And believe me, a report was written up on the lack of compassion (and probably incompetence displayed) by the representative of the mental health clinic.

Secret Shopper

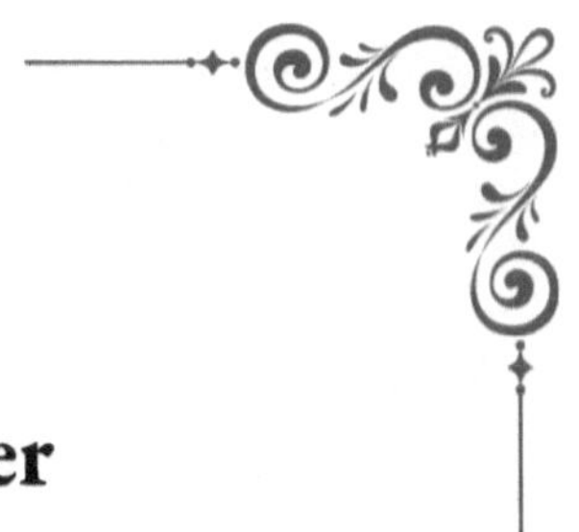

No, this was not someone who went into a clinic pretending to be a patient in order to make sure the staff was acting in the best interest of, and doing what was right for, the patient. One might think that would entail treating them with care and concern. This *could* parallel the way in which retail stores have secret shoppers that go through as a typical shopper and report on the service received. No, this was *way* more lazy than that. The VA used secret shoppers on the phone to document phone etiquette. Too bad all of the effort they placed into the *program* was wasted on most of the departments.

That *system* must've been one of the dumbest things I encountered during my time in the VA. For our clinic at least, the call usually came during the busiest times of the day. The phone would ring and myself, or another one of our staff would answer it as one should answer a phone in a place of business:

"Acute clinic, this is the (nurse or doctor, and our names) speaking, how may I help you (or how may I be of assistance)?" is how I would usually answer the phone. This way, the caller would know if they called the correct clinic as well as with whom they were speaking.

During the *secret shopper* bullshit, the statement that would usually ensue once one of our staff had answered the phone in the professional manner as indicated above, "This is your secret shopper, and you passed," and then they would usually hang up or try to get us to give them additional information.

Seriously? *What the Hell???* When we were busy, none of us had time for that *bullshit!*

I was not sure about the rest of the staff in the clinic, but as I stated, those calls usually came through during the busiest times of the day, and when I realized who it was, I would usually just hang up. I mean, after all, we were there for the patients, the Veterans, *not* to play stupid games, run by people who had no legitimate job. Reserve them for the countless clinics and ancillary services who **did not know** how to answer the phone appropriately, and still don't!

Most areas wouldn't even say which clinic or service one had reached when the phone was answered. Many times when I would phone a department I would have to verify the department or clinic as the person answering the phone did not make it initially known. I wanted to make sure I was calling the correct department or clinic. Other times, I would contact a clinic or department, wishing to speak to a specific person and would get a haughty response when the person I wished to speak to had answered the phone, but did not announce themselves and was verbally perturbed when I didn't recognize their voice. Had they announced who they were, I wouldn't have had to ask for them. Duh!

If this were such a successful program, then why when I called another clinic or other area of the building, would I receive this as a greeting?

"Hello...," and usually with an attitude.

I would wait, but when I did not hear anything after their icy greeting, I would chime in with, "Is this the so and so clinic?" or even, "Who am I speaking with?"

Or, every once in a while, when I called another clinic I would receive this type of greeting, "Such and such clinic...," and not that I was *ever* sarcastic at work, I would usually respond with, "Wonderful. And who am I speaking with?"

The responses to my questions were usually met with a very audible *sigh* from the person on the other end of the line, causing an inward smile on my end of the line. Secret shopper my ass! That program never worked properly unless they called our clinic, or maybe one or two others. Moreover, they would usually invade our patient care time, on average, once a week, with that nonsense. I'd bet that the interference was to probably to get their numbers up to make it appear as though their program was successful.

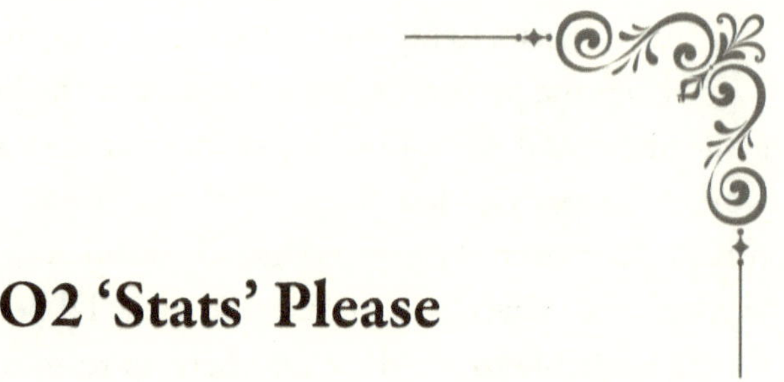

O2 'Stats' Please

"Hey ladeee", I heard, with an extremely exaggerated sugary-southern drawl, as I was charting in triage one afternoon. Attempting to finish up what I had been working on, I began to get up from my desk with the notion of heading towards the hallway. Before I was even able to exit the triage room I caught sight of an exceedingly overly made-up nurse, clothed in bright pink cartoon kitty scrubs. She stood in the doorway and excitedly spouted out, "I've got a Veteran with trouble breathing that I need y'all to see right now."

Threat to **life, limb or eyesight** are true emergencies. Difficulty breathing was usually construed as being a **threat to life**. After her outburst, I slowly rose from my chair, apologizing to the Veteran I had been currently triaging as I went, and hurried out of the triage room. I ushered Bessie to step out into the hallway, to do an *across the room triage* and get report on her patient. I fully expected to *actually see* the patient, maybe in a wheelchair, sitting in the hallway.

Okay, so if her patient was in such need of emergency treatment, why in the world did Bessie **not** bring the Veteran with her? Or rather call over, instead of wasting her time walking over to our clinic, from her primary care clinic, in order to give me report, in person, on a patient that allegedly was having trouble breathing. What she should've done was to call over and give us report if we needed to see the patient urgently. Or better yet, she should've brought the patient over with her, in a wheelchair. There seemed to be no sense of urgency from many of the staff that worked there. The primary clinic staff one time rushed over a patient with a *bunion* on their foot, asserting the need to be seen **right then and there**, but not a patient having trouble breathing. I truly did not understand.

Interestingly enough, my *boss* was walking out from the back of our clinic at that very same time and decided to listen in on our conversation. (I had to give Bertha kudos for wanting to expand her knowledge; however, I couldn't help but feel as though she was most likely just being nosey).

So, of course I had to ask, "Where is the patient?"

"He's in the clinic, Bessie huffed. "Do you want to hear his **stats**?"

Huh? It took me a half a minute to realize that she was talking about the patient's *sats* (as in oxygen **sat**uration) and not actually **stats** (as in height, weight, body composition, batting average, etc).. At her exasperated look and huffiness I couldn't help but laugh my ass off (in my head, and thought to myself that I didn't give two-shits about his *stats*. Of course I tried not to laugh out loud or look confused). Alas, I couldn't help but look at her quite perplexed. And, I did end up chuckling some and asked, "Don't you mean **sats**? I really don't care about his **stats**" (he could be 5 foot 2 inches tall and weigh 600 pounds, which would most likely account for his difficulty breathing, however that was likely **not** the issue), "but I would like to hear how his **sats** have been running."

"Are you really going to stand there and argue this with me right here and right now?" Bessie questioned.

"Yes" Bertha and I pipe in together.

(Yes, as a matter of fact I was. After all I had seen at that VA, I took any opportunity I got to teach the novice nurses I encountered. I attempted to educate them, in hopes that they might actually learn something useful to their profession.). In addition, if it had truly been an emergency, the patient should've been sitting right there in the hallway and none of this would've been an issue. Had it truly been a respiratory emergency, the Veteran would be in the clinic receiving treatment, and I would not have been standing there being given erroneous information by a *nurse* who did not know the difference between a **stat** and a **sat**.

"Yes, it's **sats**," Bertha surprising reiterated, in what could only be explained as a "Rain Man" moment (or in her case, "Rain Woman"). She actually spouted out a truly intelligent and educated response that was nothing like her usual mumbo-jumbo (hogwash).

I think I was unusually shocked speechless by that point.

"Hrmph", Bessie sighed and continued her ignorant responses. "Well, his **stats** are running in the high 80's, low 90's."

Not wanting to hold up patient care, but also wanting to make sure Bessie knew that she was incorrect in her wording. "You do realize you are saying that all wrong. It's **sat**, as in saturation of oxygen in the blood, **not** stats, as in statistics, right?"

"Are we going to continue to argue this point right here and right now?" Bessie continued to argue and completely ignore the entire fact that as an RN or an LVN, (I was really not sure what kind of schooling she completed, as she had not impressed me one bit. Basic vital signs was something one learns in Nursing 101), she should've known the difference. Especially since she supposedly had been employed in the medical field for years and allegedly performed numerous vital signs during that time, or rather should have. She should have been well aware of the obvious difference between **sats** and **stats**. In addition, where was the professionalism? Bertha and I were both trying **not** to make a *nurse* look like a total moron by continuing to spout out inappropriate terminology. Apparently, Bessie was still drinking out of the town water supply because the stupid seemed to spread through the town water supply. She didn't seem to care that she sounded ignorant as well as entirely unprofessional. (Myself, I brought my own bottled water to work, so I didn't need to drink from the local water supply.)

I DIGRESSED (ONCE AGAIN). *sigh* Knowing that our argument was futile and I was not getting through to her, I asked, "So, where is the patient?"

"Like I said, he's in the clinic."

Now with a confused look on my face I had to ask, "Why? If he's having such difficulty breathing, why did you not bring him over here in the first place?"

"I wasn't sure you all would agree to see him."

Huh? They have rushed patients over with bunions to be seen *right away*, but someone with difficulty breathing they kept in the clinic because they *thought* we may not agree to see the patient! ***WTH?*** (What the Hell?) Sometimes I wondered if some people even heard themselves talk and actually realized what was coming out of their mouths. I say this because, to the educated public, their words made no sense whatsoever.

"I, uh, can bring him over now," she stated, again, with no real sense of urgency.

"*Um, yes, please do*," I responded with just a tad bit of sarcasm and laced with *duh, WTH were you thinking*, attitude.

As Bessie walked away, heading back to her clinic to wheel the patient over to be evaluated, all I could do was shake my head as I looked at Bertha and asked, "Does she ***really*** not know what a saturation is? I mean, she's been a nurse or aide and in the medical field for some time now, right?"

"Yes, I'll have a talk with her manager," Was Bertha's simple response.

Oh, whoopdeedoo... I knew from experience how that'd go. *Can you believe my nurse embarrassed your nurse in front of me because they were mispronouncing* **sats** *as* **stats**?

When in fact the *manager* was the one who ***should've been*** educating their staff when a need arose. Somehow, from past occurrences with Bertha and Gus (the other manager), I was willing to bet that Bertha would find a way in which to blame the incident on me, purely because I was the *outsider* and not a local (born and raised) in town. Whatever! Just so long as our Veterans received the care and treatment they needed, and in a timely manner, she could **say** what she wanted. I knew the truth.

Call the Cops, He's Suicidal!

Imagine, it's close to, if not already after, 4pm, characteristically half an hour prior to the closing time for the facility and quitting time for most VA employees, on yet another Friday afternoon. I looked up from my computer, as a nurse from another clinic hurriedly escorted an ambulatory Veteran into our clinic yelling loudly to anyone that'd listen (or for everyone to hear, as other Veterans started peeking out of their cubicles to see what the commotion was all about), "Call the cops, he's suicidal."

So, of course I looked up and spied Max, one of my favorite Veterans, and watched him as he leisurely strolled into our clinic, behind the nurse. Chuckling under my breath, I asked the nurse somewhat incredulously, "Who him?" pointing at Max. "No he's not." I stated matter-of-factly, chuckling and shaking my head.

The nurse responded with, "Yes, he is. Where do you want him?" No hint of compassion at all for someone allegedly suicidal.

Rolling my eyes, I pointed to the only vacant room we had left, which just so happened to be right across from the nurse's station, indicating that they should head to that room.

I honestly could not tell if Max has an amused look on his face, or an extremely pissed-off smirk as he walked by with the nurse and into the vacant room I had just directed them towards. And,... what about HIPAA (the Health Insurance Portability and Accountability Act) – meaning... an individual's medical information is not to be made public knowledge. Or rather simple patient privacy, which the nurse was violating on an epic level, by announcing to the entire clinic what she was bringing the patient in for, in front of all the other patients as well as any staff still milling around.

Complete HIPAA/Privacy violation, as Max walked behind the nurse, and all of the other patients could be seen peeking out of their rooms to observe the commotion, the nurse was telling everyone who could hear, Max's supposed complaint. Once they passed by the nurse's station and into the one room I had indicated they go, I continued to chuckle and said, to no one in particular, "What the hell's going on now?" and continued with what I had been previously doing, most likely catching up on patient charting.

The nurse, after placing Max in the room, came up to the desk and asked, "Does anyone want report?"

I figured I'd bite, I thought as my morbid curiosity kicked in. "Sure, I'll take report. What'cha got?"

That was when the nurse tried to convince me that Max wanted to kill himself. "The doctor told me that Max is suicidal and that I should bring him over here."

"That's all you have for us?" I asked.

"Yes," she stated rather emphatically.

"Did you do anything for him?" I began, "Such as drawing any labs or any other evaluations?"

"No! The doctor said to escort him immediately over to you all."

Knowing the provider in the clinic that he had just left, as well as the nurse that practically dragged him over to us yelling out like she did, I thought that might've made him *homicidal*, but certainly not suicidal. After her abbreviated report, the nurse left our department and the cops showed up. All three officers were looking dumbfounded when one of them spoke up and asked, "We were told that you all have someone that is suicidal. Who is it?

With that, I answered truthfully, "No one."

That triggered one of the cops to blurt out, "Well that nurse from the other clinic said there's a suicidal patient here."

"Yeah, and did you notice that that nurse has also left the department? We have yet to evaluate our newest patient. As of right now, we don't have any suicidal patients," I informed them, adding in, "If we had a suicidal patient we would have either called you ourselves or had someone sitting with the patient."

The cop persisted, "Well, that nurse said that she brought a suicidal Veteran here to the clinic when she called us."

"As I just said, that nurse left and is no longer responsible for the Veteran. She unceremoniously dumped another Veteran in our laps, and no one has yet to evaluate him. Furthermore, *we* didn't call you. If you have any questions, I'd suggest you contact the person that called you and take it up with them."

Had Max truly been suicidal, the nurse should have remained with him until someone relieved her of their suicidal watch duties. Drama in the VA!

Finishing up what I had been doing, I was the first to get up and head towards Max's cubicle. I was always up for a good, juicy, story. Guess I'd have to wait another day. Once I stepped into the room that Max had been brusquely dumped into I closed the door and curtain to diminish the outside observers from peering into the cubicle through the clear glass sliding doors. Then and only then did I start my assessment. "Hey Max, what's up? Do you really want to kill yourself?" I asked more or less jokingly, rolling my eyes, as I was almost sure I knew what his answer would be.

Shaking his head chucking, out loud he said "Hell no! I have no idea what is wrong with these people. All I wanted was ... " he started to say something and his voice just softened and he put up his hands as if to say, *What can I do.* Continuing, "I got pissed off and I guess I got kinda loud over there in the clinic, and that is when the doctor said I was a threat to myself and they brought me over here."

Chuckle, chuckle, chuckle I started with a small laugh, but it was truly not more than a second before Max joined in. Before long we were both laughing our asses off.

(OKAY, A MINUTE OR SO of intermission was needed to finish laughing before the story continued. That story is still funny to this day.)

"SERIOUSLY?" I ASKED Max. "I apologize, I am definitely not laughing at you, I am laughing at the entire situation because in the short time I've gotten to know you here, you certainly do not strike me as the kind of person that wants to kill himself."

Again, we both started laughing uncontrollably and at that precise moment was when Dr. Lynn decided to join our little *party*.

As Dr. Fitzgerald had fully entered the cubicle I finally was able to compose myself enough to continue with my assessment. "Okay, tell me what's going on," I asked.

"That new doctor over there (referring to the primary care clinic) wanted to change my medications for no reason. I've been on these same medications for years and all I wanted to do was to stay on the same medicine they had me on for years, but each time the clinic changes doctors they want to change my medications and I am just freaking fed up with it and I guess I got kinda loud, and that was when the doctor said I was a threat to myself and the nurse brought me over here. Well, after this I may be a slight bit **homicidal**, but I certainly have no intention of killing myself. Sure, we all have thoughts from time to time, but I am certainly not going to act on them."

I shook my head and acquiesced with him. If someone was to say they've never had one suicidal thought, they'd be lying.

Throughout our interaction, from the time the doctor first walked into the room she listened, then after Max's last statement Dr. Lynn shook her head and walked out of the room, saying nothing. I followed, after politely excusing myself from Max, "Max, I'll be right back. Let me see what the doctor wants to do."

While talking with Dr. Fitzgerald, the primary care doctor finally decided to grace us with his presence and attempted to explain to Dr. Lynn why he sent the Veteran to us. The doctor visually struggled through his explanation, without persuading any of us, that Max was suicidal. When the doctor was done talking, I chimed in matter-of-factly (no filter around), "He's not suicidal."

The doctor looked at me like he had no idea where I had come from and then with a huff he turned back to Dr. Lynn in an attempt to convince **her** that Max was in fact was suicidal.

Once the clinic doctor left, Dr. Lynn went back into the room with Max for, I could only guess was a little tete-a-tete... She then came out, followed closely behind by Max who proceeded out of the clinic and assumedly on his way home. Nothing more to see here. Max obviously was **not** suicidal, as if he had been, Dr. Lynn would not have let him walk out on his own accord.

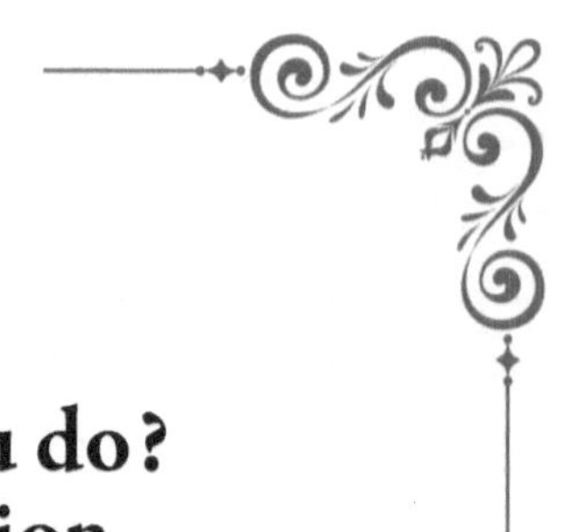

What would you do?
(With a Flotation
Device)

One of the first months of my working at the VA, I noticed that those in *leadership* seemed to have nothing more to do than to attend meetings daily and wander around the clinic oblivious to what all was happening. Oh, and those meetings occurred at least two to three times (or more) a day, every day of the week. When they weren't in a meeting, or strolling around aimlessly, they would walk around the facility and perform *inspections* (as they liked to call them) and overall seemingly **not** performing the job they were originally hired on to carry out in the first place, that of managing (or rather leading) their people. I attributed that to the simple fact most did not know *how* to perform the job of a manager or leader. Therefore, those individuals sought to generate a smokescreen in order to make the employees *think* they actually knew what they were doing. Oh how they deluded themselves. A majority of the employees knew exactly what game the *management* was struggling to play.

During one of their **many inspections**, the disaster team head, Fern, showed up in the triage room as I was preparing myself for the day ahead. First and foremost, that individual person did not appear as though she had **ever** done much *walking around the facility* doing nothing, as others in positions of *leadership* have done. Rather, it seemed more appropriate that Fern was one that would be *doing nothing period*! Of course, that was all just my personal assertions. I mentioned this because she appeared extremely short of breath when she walked into the room, probably due to her massively ample girth.

Once again, I digress.

AS THE HEAD OF THE disaster team, Fern shuffled into the room and without preamble, asked me "What would you do in the event of a disaster?"

I looked at her somewhat dumbfounded and waited for her to finish asking me the rest of the question, or at the very least, provide me with some more details. You know, part two of the question, or even a little more information so that I could've actually answered the question. I sensed that maybe with her extremely ample girth she needed additional time to get the words out fully and describe what she was trying to ascertain as far as an answer from me.

As I waited, Fern just looked at me as though waiting for an answer. I was wrong. Yep, that was the entire question. I thought to myself, *What the Fuck? Did the thought just short out in her brain and not make it out of her mouth in time? I mean, seriously, what was she thinking?*

"Um,... you're going to have to give me a little more information," I finally spat out, realizing that Fern was **not** going to offer up any more information related to her initial question.

She then just repeated her initial question, "What would you do in a disaster?"

Okay, again I contemplated the question. Fern must've seriously thought she was making sense. There were **so** many ways I could have gone with that question. Initially I tried to be polite. Notice, the operative word there was **try**.

"Okay, so are we talking a disaster in the building?" I began. Obviously I was going to have to drag the additional information from Fern.

She responded with, "No, just any kind of disaster."

Seriously! That was all the information I was going to get out of her? Okay, so I was running in downtown San Diego when 9-11 occurred. I saw blips of the incident on TVs in the shop windows. Once I got home, I got a call from a friend stationed in Japan and that's when I knew something bad was going on. I then turned on the TV and saw the disaster that had unfolded. As far as *that* particular disaster, I mourned and went about my day, as it was over three-thousand miles away in New York and I was in California. What could I really do at that point? So again, I pondered what it was that Fern was really trying to ascertain. Frankly, I was not sure she even knew herself.

For starters, it would depend on **what** type of disaster had occurred, how I would react. The VA facility was housed in a rather large building for the size of the surrounding town. If there's a fire on the complete opposite side of the building, on the top floor, and depending on the size of the fire, I would probably continue taking care of my patients and not even bat an eye, because there were *so* many other people in the building with irrelevant jobs that could assist in evacuating patients from the top floor, if needed. Of course, Fern would probably have had a hard time evacuating herself, let alone being able to help someone else. But, that was a personal problem of hers, not my concern, and one I choose not to delve into at that point in time. Okay, striving to remain calm, not smirk, roll my eyes as I tended to do when faced with stupid people who say or do ridiculous things, or downright laugh out loud, I took several deep, somewhat calming, breaths. I, once again, took a crack at dragging more information out of Fern. (Not the name I used while recounting the story with my co-workers, which was a way less *politically correct* term.)

"Okay, you're really going to have to be a little more specific here. I mean, depending on **what** kind of disaster and **where** it is will determine what I would do. So, what kind of disaster and where is this disaster you are talking about?"

"I just want to know what you would do in the case of a disaster," Fern blurted out, visibly frustrated.

*'Oh*My*God'*, seriously? And there I was, boxed into the room without access to a door ('cause Fern's ample girth was blocking the only exit **out** of the room), except to lock myself in the bathroom, which was starting to look pretty good by then. I could feign diarrhea or vomiting (or both) and hightail it into the bathroom and hope that Fern would waddle her way out of my triage room. That option was definitely worth further consideration.

Instead, I responded with, "I honestly don't know what you want from me." (That whole time I was **so** trying not to be sarcastic or condescending in the least, however, it was becoming a *huge* struggle by that time.) "If we are talking about a disaster here in the clinic, then I can give you a little information as to what I would do depending on the type of disaster. However, I **would** need to know what kind of disaster you are talking about. Fire, flood, earthquake, active shooter, hurricane, tornado, contagious outbreak... If you are talking about a disaster in the community, then you need to think about **where** the disaster is, **what** kind you are referring to, **how** it affects us here in this clinic and whether it is an earthquake, a hurricane, brush fire, plant/refinery explosion, or other type of tragedy. **What kind of disaster are you wanting me to describe** what I would do? Depending on the kind of disaster you have simulated in your head will denote how **I** would respond. I seriously need a little more information before I can answer your original question." With that, I finished my tirade and allowed her to speak. Maybe I was missing something in her initial question, but I seriously doubted that.

Why the fuck was I doing her job? Apparently, her line of questioning was not thought out past her initial query. Fern should have thought about at least some of those questions before approaching me (or anyone else for that matter) and asking such an incomplete and inappropriate, and frankly absurd, question. After all, she was the *disaster coordinator*. It was beginning to become apparent that Fern has never experienced a real-life disaster (or organized any kind of training for one) firsthand.

Without so much as a peep, Fern turned on her heel and waddled back out of the triage room and away from the clinic. Okay, guess she didn't want to delve further into the issue anymore, I reflected to myself.

ONCE FERN WAS OUT OF sight, I headed to the back of the clinic and approached my co-workers. Pondering that maybe, just maybe, I was missing something from Fern's visit and attempted at gaining some insight.

"Who's the stupid fat bitch in charge of disaster planning?" (Yeah, I think I probably did say those exact words. Remember, no filter, and I did make up her name because I really, to this day, have no freaking clue what her real name was.) Leslie, our nurse who'd been with the clinic almost from the get-go, rattled off some name, which meant absolutely nothing to me.

"Well, she's a complete and total moron," I stated plainly, and as I did, I heard Dr. Fitzgerald snickering over in the corner.

"I got a question for you," I started asking no one in particular, "What would you do in the event of a disaster?" As I posed the question to my co-workers sitting there, including Dr. Lynn, I got the deer-in-the-headlight look from **all** of them! "Phew! It wasn't *just* me thinking that question was absurd."

"Can you believe that Fern (I will using that name rather than the previous word I used to describe her) just asked me that very same question? She just asked me what I would do in the event of a disaster. That's it! Nothing else. No details, no nothing. Nada! Zilch! The *disaster* could have been on the complete other side of the clinic, or the entire other side of town, and we might never know."

As Leslie giggled, I reiterated, "I can't believe she seriously just asked me that question. I mean What the Fuck? Could she not hear what was coming out of her own mouth? No obvious connection between her pea-sized brain and her pie-hole. What would you do in a disaster? What kind of fucking question is that?" I continued my cathartic rant.

So, again I asked my co-workers, "Someone please tell me, what *would* you do in a disaster?"

After another short giggle, Leslie stated, "I have no idea, because I don't know what kind of disaster we're talking about, or where it is."

"Bingo!" I exclaimed, pointing right at Leslie. "Exactly my point! Why are these people so obtuse? And then she has the gall to look at *me*," I exaggerated as I pointed to myself, "like I have two heads when her question did not even make any sense? Ugh!!!"

After I took a few deep, somewhat calming breaths, and continued, "Okay, I'm done venting for now. I am going to back to triage and actually do my job, and hope those people stop wasting my time!"

LATER THAT DAY BERTHA came down and approached us at the nurse's station. Just to reiterate, Bertha only came to the clinic when she had something to pass on or in a pathetic attempt to reprimand us for something that we supposedly screwed up. That time was for the latter. Allegedly, according to Bertha, it was my faux pas.

"Well, we didn't do well in the disaster preparedness inspection," Bertha exclaimed rather haughtily, once she thought she had all of our attention.

Laughingly I asked, "Oh, you mean that person, Fern, who came down and asked me that stupid question? *I can't imagine why*!" (Of course I had to insert a tad bit of sarcasm into my response.)

I looked directly at Bertha and asked her the same exact question I was asked earlier that day. "What would you do in the event of a disaster?" I questioned, cocking my head to the side to gauge her reaction.

She looked at me flabbergasted. Speechless!

I waited a couple of seconds to see if she would provide any kind of answer. When she didn't, I shook my head and I exclaimed, "Exactly my point!" Which I reiterated by pointing my finger right at her "That question made absolutely no sense, at all. Now in reference to the disaster preparedness manual and its location, well, let's go back to the whole: I was not given a proper orientation. So, no I had no idea where it was, as no one showed me during my whole *orientation* process. Any further questions," I asked in a way that said that discussion was closed.

My orientation consisted of me asking all the questions I could think to find out where everything was that I might've needed or would be required to know. If I didn't think to ask the question, I would not have gotten the information that obviously was required to answer stupid questions from incompetent people. Furthermore, the VA had an excessive number of binders. If I worked there 20 years, I don't think I would've known where all of them were located or what all they encompassed. And I thought the military had a plethora of binders. At least the military had actual information in their binders. The few I **had** found at the VA only had a title page for the instruction and list of what all was purportedly included, however, no real useful information was included within the pages, like, I don't know, actual **instructions**.

In addition, my orientation consisted of me having to formulate my own orientation *go-by*/check-sheet for the computer system as I was never given any proper training on it, or where items were located in the clinic that I was supposedly required to know. Furthermore, the nurse that was assigned to *orient* me would not let me see his computer screen half the time, so to see what screens, or tabs, they were typing on.

To this day, I have no idea what that was all about, maybe he was embarrassed with his charting technique or something similar. I got tired of straining my neck over his shoulder in an attempt to see what all he was typing. So, I finally just fumbled (yes, I did use that precise word, once again, which utterly irritated Bertha and supposedly made her look bad) my way through the computer charting program, possibly screwing things up along the way.

However, I finally was able to make a guide for the charting system which I could refer back to when needed as well as pass on to my friend that started working with us a few months after I did, as well as any other incoming staff members that may have wanted to peruse through it. I wasn't all that concerned about knowing where yet *another* binder was, especially one that probably didn't contain any substantial information. I've had vast disaster training in the military and I know that those skills would've kicked in on a moment's notice should it ever come down to that. Not knowing where a particular binder was, nor reading through a specific binder, however, the point being, I never did get a proper orientation. In hindsight, an orientation checklist comprising information such as that would've been extremely helpful.

Lunch Relief

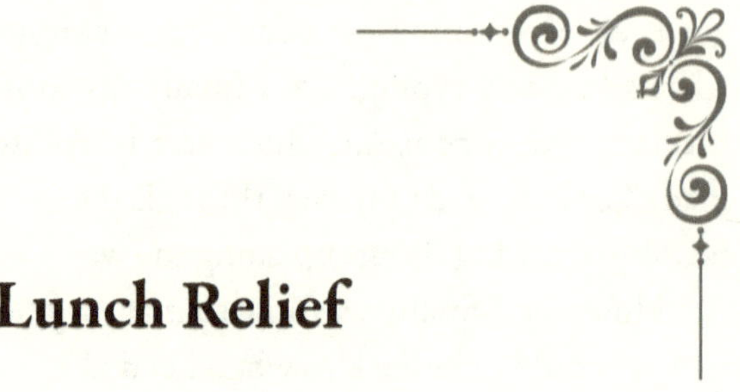

Before I explain about lunch relief, I need to explain that while working at the VA, we were scheduled for eight and a half hour days (like most forty-hour work weeks), the half hour being **unpaid** for lunch. That usually meant one would get that half hour **off** to actually, I don't know, eat lunch. Knowing I would only get paid for eight hours, albeit required to be at my job for a minimum of eight and a half hours a day, consistently longer, one would only *assume* (I know, the saying about *assuming*: it makes an ass out of you and me) that we would be allotted one half hour a day for a lunch break. **Wrong**!!! *Wrong, wrong, wrong...*

Frankly I am not sure exactly what I was thinking, as I just *assumed* that if I was not getting paid for that half an hour that it would **ultimately** be Bertha's responsibility provide coverage to ensure that her people would be allotted time for at *least* a lunch break, (especially if we were... shhhh.... **short-staffed** and were unable to relieve each other). Additionally, the union **required all** employees be allotted two, fifteen-minute breaks a day - paid (one in the morning and one in the afternoon), as well as the half hour, unpaid time away from our job location.

I could be almost positive this does not sound at all surprising to people who have somewhat normal jobs, with decent bosses (if that even existed). Oh, and if VA employees worked more than two hours overtime, there was also a requirement, by the union, to be allotted another twenty-minute paid break. I can count on one **finger** how many times *that break* happened. *Never*!!! Of course, the union was useless when it came to actually *doing* their job and standing up for their people. Pay your dues, seemed to be all they wanted of the employees, and don't cause any trouble. Hold them accountable for doing their job; you've got to be kidding!

THE PECULIAR DAY IN question was one of the countless times someone in our department requested lunch relief from Bertha. But that day we **actually received it**! I thought the walls were going to come crumbling down. That notable day she must've called in the cavalry (for that **one** specific day only). Frankly, I think Bertha was being watched and wanted to make a good impression on her *higher ups* so that they thought she was doing her job and would not realize how screwed up she really was when it came to actually *taking care of her people*.

Moving onward. One nurse, Erica, came to relieve me in triage. Funny how that day was extremely busy as we had Veterans lined up in the waiting room to be triaged and seen. In the process of giving report to my friend Erica, Bertha sidled in and, struggling to sound as though she knew what she was talking about, muttered, "Stop gossiping or you won't get your lunch break".

With my back to the door, and subsequently Bertha, Erica, and I exchanged looks like **Oh *My *God**, really? Maybe if we ignore her, she'll just go away. Bertha had taken a stab at being serious. Of course, as usual, she did not have a **clue** as to what was going on, or what needed to be done.

"Um, I'm giving turn-over and report on the patients that I know about **so that I can take a break**. That is what any prudent nurse would do when handing off care of their patients." I stated as calmly and professionally as I could muster. But, by that time, it probably had a serious air of sarcasm.

It was then quite apparent that Bertha had never done any *real* hands-on nursing *or* she has not done any in *a very long time*!!! We were taught in boot camp (as well as nursing school), "*do not leave your post until properly relieved*." Well, I guess we couldn't expect much from someone who worked *for* the VA unless they'd actually been in the military, or had a lick of common sense. Common sense seemed to be thrown OTD (out the door), or rather OTFD (out the fucking door).

After making my statement to Bertha, she just kind of stood there, shuffling from foot to foot. I could only guess it was because she obviously did not know what to do next. I glanced back at Erica and continued with my report, as we exchanged looks that could've said, *Did she really just say that? And what is she still doing here?*

Bertha was like a fish out of water in our clinic. She never really knew what to do with regards to patient care, or anything else, as far as how the clinic ran, for that matter. Although yes, she was *technically* the one *in charge* of the clinic. It was sad, really.

I FINISHED GIVING REPORT and my list of patients to be triaged next (that I knew of, as more could've signed in while Bertha was having her little hissy-fit) to Erica, along with each of their reasons for coming to the clinic. I then started out the door, when Bertha picked up a piece of fruit I had left on the desk for later when I knew I would *not* get my required afternoon break. She said to me, "Is this yours? You might want to take it or else I'll throw it away."

I grabbed the fruit and thought to myself as I walked out of the door, *Touch my fruit and I'll shove it down your throat. Leave my fucking fruit alone, and yeah, you throw it away and then we will have words. And now I freaking have to wash it **once again** since you had your grubby hands all over it'... **ewww**...*

Meanwhile, as I was taking my break, there were about three other nurses (a few *managers*) relieving our staff in the back of the clinic.

And, there are only two staff nurses actually working that day, in addition to myself. So, it took more *managers* to cover for three nurses/*worker bees* so to say. To be fair, Bertha did help out some. As a nurse, she had the knowledge and skills to be able to...

Wait for it...

Wait for it...

Hold on...

You're never going to believe it...

Have you guessed it yet?...

...remove the bedsheets between patients, and possibly wipe down the gurneys to clean them. Yep, that was it! Okay, wait, that was not entirely all. Bertha was also able to place clean sheets on the bed after cleaning it off. However, she was not able to assist in any type of nursing capacity, in the least. In fact, she couldn't even seem to function in the role of a nursing aide to keep up with vital signs, or administer simple medications.

BACK TO THE BREAKROOM. As the three of us were sitting there eating lunch we discussed the absurdity of the turn of events. In fact, we actually had the room to ourselves that day. The only people that typically used our break room were the providers from the other clinics. On the rare chance that we actually got a break, we were barely afforded the luxury of actually being able to utilize our ***own*** break room, Of course, we all sat at the table, ensured the door to the break room was closed so that we could not be overheard or spied upon, as the *managers* have been known to do.

"Holy cow, can you believe they brought so many people down to relieve us? What's that all about?" I asked aloud to no one in particular.

Continuing to contemplate out loud, I went on to say, "Oh wait. I know. It's Friday. No one here actually has a job to do. So, all of the *managers* came down here to see what the fuss was all about. And then, they made others, who actually have jobs to do, cover for us so that we can all take a lunch. Was that to try to make us feel bad?"

"Yeah right. Why are they all so stupid?" Leslie chimed in.

"That's a very good question. Unfortunately, I don't have an answer for you," I acknowledged, while Markus (the other nurse we were working with) remained quiet. He just ate his lunch in relative peace. Probably because he was the spy for Bertha, as he was her favorite and all, and was not one to cause waves, or even ripples.

We all took our time eating. Yet we felt slightly guilty for having others take time out of their busy schedules to cover us for breaks simply because the *managers* did not have the experience or competence to provide that relief themselves. Nor did they have the inclination to actually be able to relieve us on a regular basis. I think they actually believed this *show of force* put them in a good light for us to not ask for lunch breaks again. **Wrong**!

Alas, this was the **only** time that we actually received full coverage for an appropriate lunch break. I honestly think there might've been some people from the *higher echelon* visiting our VA for the day and **none** of the *managers* wanted to appear as though they were not taking care of their people. Besides, I think the *managers* needed something to do to keep themselves busy so to appear to visiting *leadership* as though they actually had a job and the supervising *leadership* wouldn't ask too many questions. If they were to ask questions, leadership might subsequently find out that middle *management* didn't actually have a job to do, or if they did, know what that job encompassed, as well as how to accomplish it.

Sadly, as I stated, this lunch relief happened only **once** in the time in which I was employed at the VA. From that day on, when we were not afforded any breaks, we were forced to add in an extra half an hour onto our already, almost daily, standard one-half to two or more hours of overtime each day, to account for the lack of a break. Of course, that never did make up for the fact that we were usually bone tired by the time we had left each day.

At one time, Bertha actually did email/text us back and carbon-copied her boss who (as they were just as ignorant) stuck up for our boss. This supervisor stated that it was our responsibility to break ourselves. *And how were we supposed to do that when, oftentimes, there were only two nurses on for the day and we had to keep two nurses on the floor at all times?* Hmmm, there was effective *management* at its best. I was always under the premise that a good manager or leader would:

1. Take care of their people,

2. Not ask someone to do something that they themselves would not do, and,

3. Know (at least a smidgen) what the job was, of the people they supervised. Leaders/managers do not necessarily have to know what all goes into the job function of their subordinates, but they **should** have some kind of working knowledge of what their employees are required to do. Additionally, as a nurse, first and foremost, a nurse **manager** should definitely be able to function as a basic nurse. I guess I was taught in a different school of leadership.

From the examples I've seen at the VA, the object is to ignore your people (unless they do something wrong and when that happens strive to slam them against the wall – not literally) and hope they make you look good. A good leader/manager would earn the appreciation of their employees. So, we took care of ourselves in the end. We added a half hour on to our overtime slip each and every day we did not get a break. And, of course, the *higher-ups* bitched, moaned, and complained about all the overtime. **Really**? There seemed to be no making them happy. Where was the sense I ask you?

What's Is Your Job Anyway?

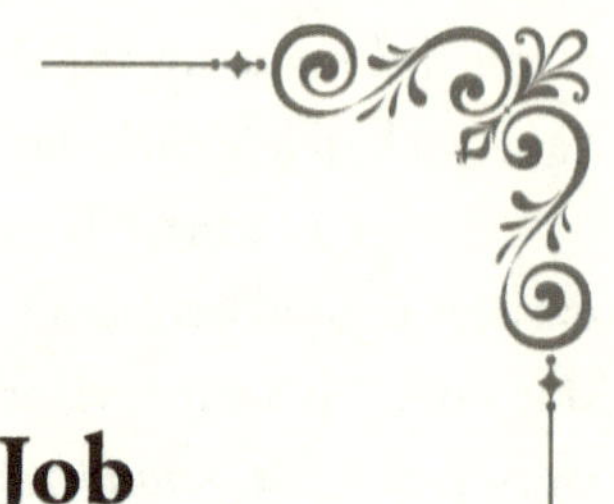

Only about a month or so into my stint at the local VA my co-workers and I were *blessed* to be working with yet another doctor, who at the time, it was questionable as to whether she actually finished her residency. Numerous rumors floated around about that topic the whole time I worked there. Based solely on her performance as a *medical provider* and *professional,* it was my humble opinion that Dr. Su Lin *never did* finish her residency. If she did, I'd say it was probably bought and paid for by *daddy,* or even the American taxpayers. It could be conceived that her residency, however stalled previously, was continued and possibly even completed at the VA. In line with this belief, it was also my humble opinion that Dr. Lin struggled to act in the role of a *competent* medical provider. By allowing the Veterans to believe that, she was a full-fledged licensed provider, when in fact she was most likely performing the position of a resident.

Regardless of when or even if Dr. Lin completed her residency, her work displayed during my employ, was that of a graduate medical doctor, at best! However, holding a degree stating, "Doctor of Medicine" does not necessarily make someone automatically intelligent or competent. Nor does that title give someone free reign to act ignorant, oh wait, I meant act superior.

As it happened, when I am surrounded by idiots, I tend to digress.

IN AN ATTEMPT TO BREAK the ice, and being new to the VA, I liked to try and get to know the people with whom I worked, in addition to where they were from. I started a conversation with Dr. Lin, by asking her, "Where are you from?" As I knew she was not from the United States, with her appearance as well as her accent.

"Nepal." She answered and then proceeded to ask haughtily, "Do you know where that is?"

"Yes. I know where that is," I responded. That's what I got for trying to be nice, and interested in my co-workers

She apparently felt the need to continue with, "And it's **not** India."

With that unnecessary response, I just looked at her with a *well, duh!* expression on my face. How freaking ridiculous. She was the one rumored to not have finished medical residency, and she was questioning *my* geographical skills. Really???

As luck would have it, Dr. Su Lin was instructed to work with us in the clinic. The doctor we worked with my first week in the clinic, Dr. Michael Dumassé, liked to make an effort at treating his medical staff (mainly nurses) as though we were his personal lackeys, and below him on the food chain. I attempted to inform Dr. Dumassé **several** times that we were **not** his secretaries, and if that was what he wanted, then he needed to go back up to his office and have his personal secretary complete those jobs he was trying to get medical professionals to perform. However, the jobs Dr. Dumassé was usually asking the nurses to complete were way above the paygrade of a secretary. Also, even as nursing or other medical professionals, we were not legally allowed, nor required, to enter orders in for the doctors, *especially* medication orders. However, Dr. Dumassé seemed to think that it was more than okay.

For the most part we were intellectually able to perform those tasks; still, it was not in our scope of practice and therefore if there had been an incident, legally we would be held responsible for our actions and accountable to the Director of Nursing. I worked hard for my nursing license and was **not** about to allow a cocky doctor (albeit a stupid one) put me in that position! All so that he could be lazy and not do his job, as the patient load was not all that strenuous. Sadly, he seemed to think he was way more important than he truly was.

Nevertheless, no matter how many times we **informed** Doctor Dumassé, who was later placed in the position with some pretentious and totally inappropriate title, in my opinion – (notice I said that he was **placed** in that position, not that he **earned** that position), he continued his exasperating attempts to utilize us as secretaries. Dr. Dumassé would come into the clinic, dictate orders and wonder why we didn't either start transcribing those order or immediately jump up to complete said orders. I was in the Navy and Air Force, **not** the Marines – don't think he's going to tell me to jump and I'd ask, 'how high'.

I told Dr. Dumassé numerous times that we were only to take verbal orders in the event of a true emergency. In those extremely rare instances, we would in fact fulfill verbal orders, so long as they were legit. But, working in a clinic, and not an Emergency Room, we were rarely faced with true *emergencies*, and therefore were not required (or even legally allowed) to take verbal orders on a regular basis. One noteworthy reason for this was the fact that Dr. Michael Dumassé (as well as others I've encountered over the years) liked to change their minds after the fact. For instance, when a verbal order did not elicit the appropriate or desired response, it was common for some doctors to say, *I never ordered that!* and then who's ass ends up on the line? Ours. No. Thank. You!

No matter how many times we articulated this to Dr. Dumassé, he never seemed to be able to grasp that fact in his oblivious mind. This was also part of the reasoning why when Dr. Lin would cover the clinic for Dr. Dumassé we had problems with her also *wanting* us to enter her orders. In a sense, basically doing her job. I kept wanting to tell her to shit in one hand and want in the other and see which one filled up first.

Some days I felt as though I was banging my head against the wall by even talking with either of those two *doctors*. Seriously, how many times can someone say *Do your job and I'll do mine*, before it may sink in? It wasn't not rocket science to be able to enter one's own orders and do the job they were hired to do. Especially at the sum of over two-hundred thousand dollar-a-year salary.

IT ALL CAME TO A HEAD one day when Dr. Lin started barking out orders and was visibly **shocked** that we were not all jumping at her beck-and-call to perform **her** job. In fact, we all just kind of looked at her like, *Please be quiet, we're trying to work here;* and, *Who do you think you are talking to?* Again, you do your job, and we'll do ours. I informed her (yet again) that we would complete the orders once they were entered and signed off in the computer. As none of our patients were emergent, so there was no reason for her to spout out, and us to carry out verbal orders.

On one particular day in question we had a variety of *talent* in the clinic; there was the MD (Medical Doctor), a FNP (Family Nurse Practitioner), a RN (Registered Nurse) and a LVN (Licensed Vocational Nurse). After several times of us, the nursing staff (and I am sure especially myself), refusing to enter orders on Dr. Lin's behalf, she approached me and Leslie asking, "If you are not entering my orders for me, then what are you doing?"

Really, did she really just ask me that question?

Without hesitation or forethought, I spouted out, "Seriously?" See, no filter. "I'm doing my job!" I wanted to add, *Duh*. "I have my own job, my own scope of practice, as does Leslie here," I said pointing next to me, "who is a LVN, and Teresita there," I made it obvious who I was referring to on the other side of the nurse's station, "is a Nurse Practitioner with her own scope of practice. We all have our own, individual, scopes of practice, as do you. **My job** is **not** to do your job and enter *your* orders for you. That is *your* job. *My job* is to carry out those orders entered by you, just so long as they are appropriate. I also have other duties in my job description." Well, that certainly did *not* go over well with Dr. Lin. I was sure that was *not* what she wanted to hear!

"Hrmph! I still don't believe that your job is not to enter my orders. Doctor Dumassé said that was your job. I mean, after all, all you're all doing is sitting here."

Biting my tongue and trying to keep from laughing and then lashing out and reaching over the counter and smacking her upside the head, I turned my head, smiled to myself, and to Leslie who was sitting next to me, and took a calming deep breath.

Finally somewhat composing myself, I turned back towards Dr. Lin and stated, "Seriously? Is that *really* what you think? I have been sitting here entering notes and assessments on *our* patients. That was until you came up and interrupted us with your ludicrous accusation. My job as an RN is *not* to do your job. That includes you entering your own orders into the computer. That is *your* job to do after assessing the patients."

"*Well*!" She huffed out, "I am going to talk to Doctor Dumassé about this. This is not right! You are supposed to be entering my orders."

Not being able to hold back anymore, I laughingly said somewhat flippantly, "Good luck with that." and waved her off to go do her job. I then turned my attention back to typing up my assessments. My *filter* just could not hold back the sarcasm any longer.

I looked at Leslie, and neither one of us could believe that Doctor Lin actually had the audacity to think that we were her lackeys. Both of us seemed to be having a difficult time holding back our laughter at the craziness of it all.

Laughter finally subsided I murmured, "Well, I guess I should contact Bertha and give her a *heads up* that this will be escalated. What the Hell was Doctor Lin thinking? *Was* she thinking? Maybe if she entered her own orders she might actually learn something. I think that's a lot of the problem. The people who are supposed to be in charge don't know what they are doing and expect us, the *trench* nurses to bail them out, all the time. It was as bad as when I first got here and I was fumbling my way through the whole computer system (I said motioning to the computer in front of me) trying to figure out what I had to document so that my charting would be complete. That was bad enough. I don't need to worry about doing the doctor's job too."

"Craziness I tell you," Leslie stated before we both broke out in fits of laughter once again. By that time, Doctor Lin was in a patient's room with the door closed.

Bertha ended up coming to the clinic (remember I mentioned she only showed up when she had to pass on some useless information, or in a pathetic attempt at reprimanding us) and spoke to Doctor Lin. Of course, Doctor Lin still refused to believe that we were not there to be her minions. Apparently she was not satisfied with the conversation she had with Bertha. So, she elevated the matter in her own way. She apparently was not too happy with the results of that outcome either.

(I may have been considered a bitch at times. But if someone had put forth the effort to do their job to the best of their ability, I would cover their ass. Then again, I would *not* do that if someone was going to be a jackass to me and just expect me to do their job, simply because they were too lazy to do it themselves!)

Later on that day, we had a little *pow-wow* with Dr. Lin, myself, the Nurse Practitioner Teresita, Bertha and Gus, the *manager* of the clinic where Dr. Lin generally worked. There were also some other busy-bodies who, to this day, I have no idea who they were or what their jobs really entailed. In that little *encounter*, Dr. Lin lied completely out of her ass. She tried to change around and cover up what she said. Once I related my side of the story she again lied and stated she said nothing of the sort. *Really*, where was her accountability and responsibility for her own actions? Oh right, there *were* none at the VA. Funny though, Teresita backed me up and agreed that what I said she also had witnessed. So, Doctor Lin had to concede to being the liar she was faulted for being.

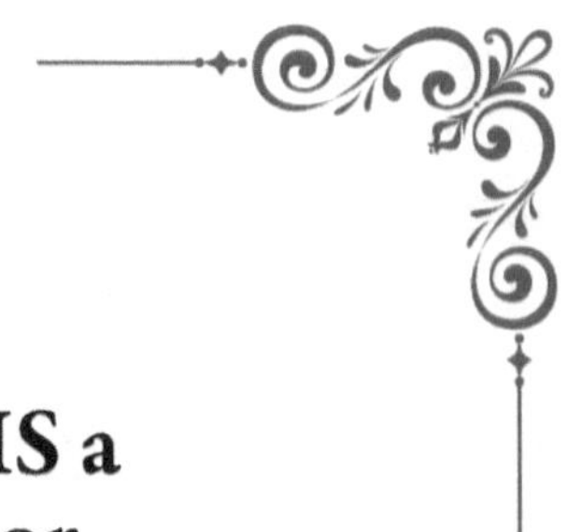

A Psychiatrist IS a
Medical Doctor

On one ***very rare*** occasion when we were slammed with patients in the clinic (oops, that was in fact more complete and utter sarcasm), we had yet another Veteran who needed a Mental Health evaluation to determine if he was in need of inpatient psychiatric treatment, or if he could be discharged home to follow-up on an outpatient basis. The Veteran presented to our clinic (or rather presented to our clinic ***after*** he left the Mental Health clinic because they refused to see him.) with depressive issues. It was another Friday afternoon, before a holiday weekend, and the staff in the Mental Health clinic apparently wanted to leave early for the holiday weekend. Unfortunately, as seemed to be the norm for their staff, one of their providers would not evaluate, or even look at, any patient until the patient was medically cleared. Medical clearance, for them, meant that ***no*** drugs or alcohol, of any amount, was in the Veteran's system. Additionally, the Veteran would need to be *medically stable* to be seen for any mental health issues (that meant no medical reasoning could be found that may have been causing the mental issues for their depression).

As was par for our clinic, we were extremely busy, as it was the end of the day and before a long weekend, and holding off other more critically ill Veterans, all the while waiting for lab results for the depressed Veteran, would've bottlenecked our entire clinic. And he couldn't be placed in the waiting room, out of sight, because if he was truly suicidal, then he might elope – escape without anyone knowing that he had in fact left the building. If that were to happen, it would make the staff responsible for his well-being in case he tried to harm himself, or worse. The reason I even mentioned that this day was a very *rare occurrence* for our clinic was that Dr. Dumassé, the Chief of Staff [or rather Acting Chief of Staff or Acting Clinic Director or whatever pretentious title he had been given (or gave himself) – as there seemed to never be any one person of authority that remained at the facility for any length of time], more or less forced the Psychiatrist to physically present himself to our clinic in order to evaluate *their* patient. Regardless of the fact that it was probably around three or four o'clock on a Friday afternoon, of a holiday weekend when everyone decided to take a long weekend.

The Psychiatrist, Dr. Xander Krupski, most likely would have been more than happy to have been able to slink out of the clinic early, like most everyone else, to start his holiday weekend sooner. Yet, Dr. Krupski arrived in our clinic surprisingly stealthy as his size denoted that he shouldn't be able to do anything very discreetly. He sidled up to the nurse's station, seemingly attempting to become an actual part of said nurse's station, as he struggled to blend right into it. All the while, he appeared more than perturbed at being called away from his early exodus from the clinic for the weekend.

"Um, can someone please tell me what I am doing here?" Dr. Krupski announced to no one in particular. We all just kind of looked at each other. I looked around because I had no idea who he was. It wasn't as though mental health providers were frequent fixtures in our clinic. And I had absolutely no idea who Dr. Krupski was, nor did I even know what he looked like.

Our provider at that time, Doctor Fitzgerald, turned slowly around, clearly irritated at the interruption and the fact that she now had to explain to yet one more doctor about how to care for their own patients.

"Yes, well I have four patients in the clinic at this time, and another six waiting to be seen. We have one of yours down in the end room (she said, pointing to direct Dr. Krupski towards the appropriate room) who needs a mental health clearance and determination for further treatment."

"Are their labs back yet?" Questioned Doctor Krupski.

"I have no idea. I'm busy with a cardiac patient, as well as one with difficulty breathing. Frankly, that one is not high on my list of priorities at this time. You are more than welcome to go check on *your* patient."

"Well, I can't wait around all evening, I have to get home," he spouted out, oblivious as to how insensitive his whining fell on deaf ears.

Seriously? Did Dr. Krupski really just have the gall to say that, right there in front of our entire clinic staff that rarely, if *ever*, got to leave on time, let alone *early*? Didn't we all need, or want to get home?

"Well, if you want to find out the results you can either look them up in the computer or call the lab. I am extremely busy at this time and frankly I do not have time to hold your hand to do your job, as well as mine," Stated Doctor, Lynn, rationally.

"How can I look them up on the computer, my computer is upstairs on the 3rd floor?" Doctor Krupski whined.

What a complete and utter moron. All the computers in the whole clinic, 1st through 5th floors were set up the same. Anyone could log into just about any computer, in any area of the clinic, and access charts that they have access to in their own office. There were at least two available computers for Doctor Krupski to access the information he needed to be able to (assumingly) competently perform his job.

"Hrmph!" Doctor Fitzgerald practically grumbled and turned her chair around, getting back to the charts she was working on before the oh so rude interruption.

So, Doctor Krupski, continued to stand at the end of the nurse's station counter looking lost as though he has no clue on how to proceed. I would've been willing to bet a lot of money that he was never in the military, not only because of his ample size, however, that would've been a big clue, but mainly because of his complete inability to adapt to a new situation and just roll with it. Hence, *Semper Gumby*.

Of course, I couldn't hold back as usual and me and my big mouth chimed in, "There are two computers right there (pointing to the open and available computers) that you can use. You *do* have your ID card, right?" It wasn't uncommon for providers, or other staff with their own offices to leave their ID card in their computers when they left for the evening. Although that was not policy, or supposedly allowed, it still happened. Of course, I had **never** seen that firsthand. Ha! That seemed to happen all the time.

As it turned out, Bertha was also called down, and grudgingly presented to the clinic. Again, it was the end of the day on a Friday evening, before a holiday weekend, and everyone wanted to go home early and dump their remaining patients on our clinic staff. By that time we were at the peak of patient care and Doctor Fitzgerald was busy with four other highly acute Veterans which either needed transportation for transfer to a higher level of care, or needed to be discharged home so that she could see the other six Veterans waiting patiently to be seen for their urgent complaints.

Doctor Krupski, who was well known for his flamboyant nature as well as his theatrics when it came to *actual* patient care, spent the better half of an hour whining about why he was called down to our clinic when the Veteran was not yet medically cleared for evaluation by a Mental Health provider. Myself, Bertha, the Acting Chief of Staff or Acting Clinic Director (I still, had no idea what title he was using), and Doctor Krupski then proceeded into the triage room for the psychiatrist to continue his theatrics, away from the patients.

"I cannot evaluate a Veteran until they are medically cleared to be seen," Doctor Krupski whined.

"Any competent medical doctor can evaluate a patient for medical clearance and for inpatient treatment. And I do believe a psychiatrist falls into that category. Isn't a psychiatrist a medical doctor first and foremost?" I began the conversation quite innocently, or rather an effort of an attempt at innocence. Yep, once again, no filter. Shit just seemed to slip out. Yeah, Doctor Krupski did not like that one bit. Ooops, I guess he should've paid more attention in medical school and his internship.

"Yes, a psychiatrist if fully able to medically clear a Mental Health patient for inpatient treatment," Bertha chimed in. (Whoohoo! Chalk up another point for Bertha). Meanwhile, the Acting Chief of Staff just stood there shaking his head, and chuckling, in concurrence. After all, what **could** he have said, especially when he knew what we had stated was true? That was just one of the very rare occasions which made me pleased that Bertha actually stood up for her people.

At that, Doctor Krupski just fumed and paused for a moment. If I had to guess, it was because he was not entirely sure **what** to do at that point. After his brief pause, Doctor Krupski then replied, "Oh, well that's fine! But, I am not entirely sure how to evaluate and interpret the lab results."

Really?!?!? Are you fucking kidding me? A clerk could tell if there were, at the very least, drugs or alcohol in the Veteran's system. Also, if the labs were out of range, as it specified on the read-out itself. But I digress.

And again, with the no filter, "But aren't you a Medical Doctor?" I pushed the issue because I just couldn't seem to help myself on that account. That was a mix of no filter and **Oh*My*God**, seriously, do your fucking job for once in your life!

With a look that I figured he'd like to think could make the floor swallow me up, muttered whining again, "But I haven't practiced medicine in a very long time."

And...that's my fault how? Oh well, that's on him. Guess he should've kept up on his skills because one never knows when they might be needed.

That entire exchange explained *so* much with regards to having any Mental Health provider voluntarily agree to actually evaluate and medically clear their own patients. I honestly did not think it was entirely because they didn't want to see their patients, although I do believe that **was** a large part of it. After that interaction, I firmly believed that the lack of Mental Health providers willing to see their own patients was probably due in part to the fact that they were like fish out of water when it came to actual face-to-face interaction with the Veterans.

Not knowing how to relate to Veterans in their own way put the Mental Health providers at a huge disadvantage. I was not giving them a pass **by any means**. I am merely stating the most probable cause of their lack of proper care related to Mental Health the Veterans received. One reason why Mental Health providers would be best at treating Veterans if they, themselves had served in the military. That way they would be able to better relate to the past experiences of Veterans.

After that encounter however, Doctor Krupski proceeded to somehow fumble through evaluating his patient and eventually provided a disposition. That included asking the clinic staff how to go about transferring a patient to a facility that accepted inpatient Veterans. It was a start. I'd give him that. Unfortunately, all the effort placed into that one incident, did not last past the weekend. It was an almost constant struggle to have Mental Health evaluate their own patients. Their staff gave the impression that they would do **whatever** they could to get anyone else to evaluate those Veterans.

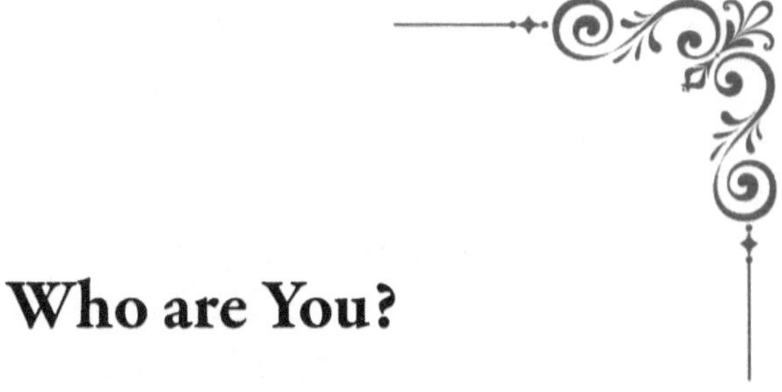

Who are You?

Several years after resigning my position at the local VA I decided to use my time and volunteer at that very same VA, seeing as they were not banging down the doors to rehire me. My goal was to hang out with the guys that are stuck there as inpatients. Again, I was a glutton for punishment. But that time the *higher-ups* really didn't have control over me, as I was volunteering my time and obviously not getting paid, yet they tried however unsuccessfully. Unfortunately, it took countless months to get approval to volunteer. Honestly, I had no idea what the problem was. My history and experience should've allowed me the chance to begin sharing my time right away.

Apparently, the so-called *powers that be* had other ideas. I was getting cut off at every avenue I took towards volunteering. Finally, I was introduced to the Public Affairs Officer, Shaneka Alton, who was, at the time, in charge of the volunteers. One day, when I just so happened to be in the clinic for an event, I approached her and asked, "I heard you were in charge of the volunteers. What do I need to do or who do I need to talk to in order to get this going?"

As was par for most of the employees at the VA, tactlessly she rudely responded with a question, "And who are you?"

"My apologies. I am Lila Tarankowski. I've spoken with Caleb up in the volunteer office and was told I need to get an ID card, but I have yet to get the appropriate paperwork signed to make that happen."

"Okay," she started with a haughty air of superiority, "follow me to my office, I am late for a meeting."

We walked to the other side of the building and once arriving in her office, she said, "Let me write your name and phone number down here and I will get back to you tomorrow regarding the form for your ID."

I supplied her the requested information and she jotted it down on a tablet on her desk. I then thanked her and left her office. I fully expected to hear from her the following day, as she made a point to tell me that she would call.

Three days later I had still not heard back from Ms. Alton. I figured I'd wait a little longer to see if she'd call me like she said she would, albeit late. About a month after our first encounter I returned to the VA as I had an appointment. By chance I ran into (almost literally) none other than Ms. Shaneka Alton.

"Oh hey," I started nonchalantly, and attempted to remain oblivious to the fact that she had not called me. "What have you heard about the form for my ID card?" I asked innocently.

She looked at me as though she had never seen my face before and asked, "Who are you?"

Trying not to laugh at the absurdity as well as her incompetence at performing her job I said matter-of-factly, "I am Lila Tarankowski. We spoke a month ago about me volunteering. You were going to call me back the day after we spoke and I never heard back."

"What? I don't know what you are talking about," she started as though I was a moron. "Oh wait, I remember you. Yes, I was going to call, but didn't find out anything about the form for the ID card."

Pushing the issue as usual I stated, "You said you were going to call. I expected a call. When someone tells me they'd do something, I expect them to follow through. If you didn't have the information, the *least* you could've done would have been to call, like you said you would, and inform me of that fact. Where are you now with getting that accomplished?" I asked, determined to hold her accountable for doing what she said she would.

"I'll work on that and get back to you," she started...

I eyed her with a looked that said I don't believe you, could you blame me?

"Really, I will get back to you this time. Once I find out what all I need to get you started volunteering."

"I'm gonna hold you to that." With that I walked away and out of the building.

A FEW WEEKS LATER I still had not heard back from Ms. Alton, but I did receive an email from Caleb informing me that I could show up at his office and pick up the form to obtain my volunteer ID. Simple as that. I still was not sure what all the hold-up was in the first place, with Ms. Alton.

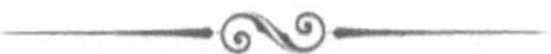

SEVERAL WEEKS OF VOLUNTEERING and creating *havoc* with the old men in the nursing home I had the *lovely* opportunity to run into Ms. Alton, yet again. That time I actually had one of my *charges* with me as we were traversing the halls of the VA and creating more havoc. After all, what did Marines do but cause trouble. We were actually observing a small ceremony for Veterans Day. Shaneka sidled up to me and spoke into my shoulder (she was quite short).

"I am going to need a schedule from you of the days and times you'll be here in the building," she started.

"No you don't," I simply responded.

"Well, I need to know ahead of time when you're going to be in the building," she pushed.

"No you don't," I repeated.

Stuttering she tried again, "Well, we need to know when you'll be here so that we can have something worthwhile and rewarding for you to do as a volunteer."

I could tell she was attempting to make me feel as though she cared about my volunteer experience, when in fact I knew she was just being nosey and wanting to know when I would be in the building, period. "No you don't," I repeated again. "I already have something to do that is quite rewarding." And I did. I truly enjoyed hanging out with my fellow Vets and of course causing trouble, not really (the causing trouble part).

"We still need to know what days you're going to be here," she persisted.

So, I tried to placate her, if only to shut her up about the issue. I was a volunteer, and therefore was there on *my* time, whenever I might've been available. "I will be here weekly one day a week, unless something comes up."

"Well, if you're not going to be here, then we need to know twenty-four hours in advance," she stated as though she had the upper hand in our conversation.

What the Fuck? Employees could call-in sick the morning of when they were supposed to work and a freaking volunteer needed to let you know a day early. I called bullshit on that. Again I felt my previous statement was appropriate and responded easily with, "No you don't."

Stuttering, she tried again, "Ye..., yes....Yes we do."

Thinking to myself and wanting to spout out loud, *No, you want to know when I'll be in the building so that you can either hide anything that I might see of wrongdoing or so you can just hide from me, or keep tabs on what I was doing.* Instead I cut her off at the pass, telling her flat out, "I am a volunteer, I am not an employee. I am not getting paid for my time and so I will be here *when* and *if* I have the time to volunteer. As far as if I cannot make it one week, then I will not be here. There is absolutely *no reason* I need to give you twenty-four hours' notice if I am not showing up. Employees can call-in sick two hours before the start of their shift. Why would a volunteer be held to more stringent regulations? I will be here when I have the time. If something comes up,

I will be in contact with Caleb. Do you have any further questions?" I asked.

Again stuttering and grumbling incoherently, Ms. Alton did not press the issue further.

"Good, because I have to get Mr. Joseph here back to his floor for lunch. Have a good day." With that, I wheeled Mr. Joseph out of the conference room and back to his floor.

Part II
The Veterans

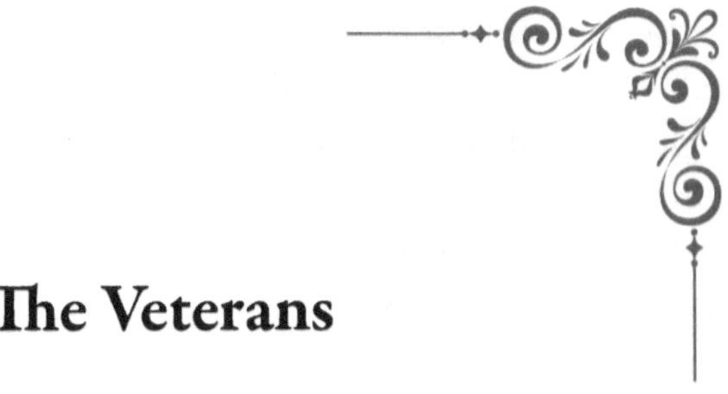

The Veterans

Veterans are not without their own comedy, drama or personal issues. Like in the civilian world, Veterans also have access to medical websites, some reputable and some not so much, as well as other not so respectable sites touting medical information, like faux news and information outlets. Some Veterans choose to utilize this avenue quite often, thus making for comedic relief on days in which it was so dearly needed by the staff, as well as other Veterans. On the contrary, not all of the following stories are comedies. In fact, some of the patients I've written about are Veterans who were either not well cared for by the staff at the VA or they are Veterans whose medical issues have been caused by staff that were less than competent.

The following pages are several examples of these types of Veterans. The Veterans I have chosen to write about have become near and dear to my heart. They have either been blatantly ignored or brushed aside by the very people that had taken an oath and sworn to care for them. For the staff members that had pledged to place the care of these Veterans first and foremost, their loyalty to their duty has been considerably deficient. Oftentimes those staff members had been overheard stating, *That's not my job* or *I don't know **what** they're complaining about* and even *They can come back later*. Unfortunately, a majority of those employees have conveniently forgotten the affirmation they pledged when they first were hired on at the VA.

The remaining stories have been included for comic relief and to show that patients in the VA system were no different than patients in the civilian world. After all, people are people, and someone once told me that the people in the military have to come from somewhere, right? The other stories are about Veterans that were simply available to us (myself and my co-workers), most likely not by their own choosing, to lighten the mood during some of our busiest and often most trying days.

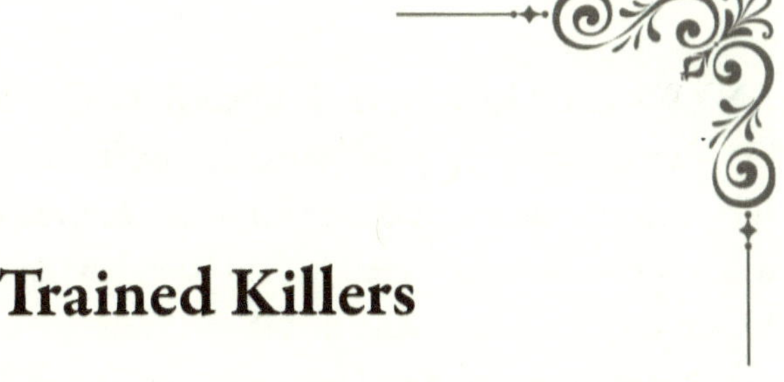

Trained Killers

Joe was your typical all-American guy who chose to join the military right out of high school. During his four-year enlistment his dedication and bravery earned him the loving nickname G.I. Joe. For the most part, the Army was known for their soldiers/grunts routinely performing grueling training and ruck-marches, oftentimes having to carry upwards of 70 or more pounds on their backs in order to complete those extended marches. Being the macho guy he was (as many young men were during that time), Joe *walked off* most of his injuries after separating from the Army. Almost ten years later, and well into his thirties, Joe started having issues with his knees from the grueling training completed in the Army over a decade prior. He never felt the need to utilize the VA health care facility previously, but decided it was finally time.

DURING THE FIRST MONTH or so that I worked at the VA there happened to be a new Nurse Practitioner training in our clinic, under the doctor from hell, Dr. Dumassé. I had wanted to call him, Doctor Satan, however, that would most likely be considered politically inappropriate or incorrect, and so I have dubbed him Dr. Michael Dumassé. Either way, that was the doctor who's been in several previous stories and who thought we are all his minions, and no, I'm not talking about the short little yellow type of *minions* from the movies.

ANYWAY, EARLY ONE MORNING G.I. Joe came in to be seen for worsening knee pain, most likely from carrying 50-70+-pound rucksack around in the desert for weeks or even months at a time. As he was in his thirties he stated he had been having the issue for some time. When further questioned, he informed me he wanted to get it checked out before it became a real issue for him. He told me he had the pain for the last four years of his enlistment or so, but was unable to do anything about it or he'd have been placed in a desk job. So he suffered through the pain during his ruck-marches and jumping out of helicopters and airplanes, and whatever else was required of him. Most people I've met in the military, if they were in active type jobs, did not want to be glued to a desk purely due to an injury.

Working six days a week, Joe did not have much free time and therefore showed up one day in our clinic. When I went into the room to assess him, I asked why he had not presented his issue to his primary care doctor as it had been going on for years.

Joe responded with, "I have had appointments scheduled over the last several months that I would show up for, only to find out that they were canceled for one reason or another by the VA staff, most of which I didn't find out about until I showed up for the appointment. It was becoming a burden on me because I would take off half a day from work to show up for an appointment, only to be told that my appointment had been canceled. Before today, the last one was about a week or so ago, with the same response, they told me 'we apologize, but your doctor is not here today. Didn't anyone contact you about this?' I told them that was not the first time that the VA had canceled my appointment and hadn't even contacted me. So, I missed a whole day of work already today, and I can't afford to miss another day like that, and so that they'll maybe give me some Motrin to take for the pain. I want to find out what is going on with my knee and get it fixed. If I take off another whole day anytime soon then I will lose my job."

Shaking my head I concurred, "I totally understand." I had no qualms in seeing Joe, as that was what the VA was there for and more importantly what our clinic was there for, to pick up the slack from the other clinics that, for one reason or another, were unable (or unwilling) to care for their own Veterans.

He continued with, "I know I should've been seen previously for the pain but, I've been working six days a week and this is the first time I've had a day off during the week and this has been my earliest chance to really get it looked at."

"No problem, when was the last time you had x-rays done on it, or a CT?" I asked.

"If I had x-rays done it's been years. Probably before I got out of the military."

"Well, I'll talk to the doctor, at least we'll order an x-ray because they won't do a CT or MRI until you've had baseline x-rays done recently, and it sounds like it's been a while since you've had any imaging done. I'll go start on that and find out when the doctor will be in to see you."

"Thank you, ma'am," he sounded relieved that he might actually get some treatment.

Before I got up and leave the cubicle G.I Joe was in, Dr. Dumassé arrived with his huge haughty attitude in tow, followed by the new Nurse Practitioner, Teresita. I was sitting on the gurney talking eye-to-eye with Joe. He was sitting on the chair across from me, and when Dr. Dumassé came in he leaned against the wall, and began to assumedly *teach* Teresita how to question a patient. Apparently his line of questioning included pausing between each question asked. (To me, it seemed as though he had no idea what he should be asking, and therefore paused, searching for questions with which to ask, or possibly waiting for the Veteran to self-diagnose.)

Joe's gaze shifted from the Dr. Dumassé and Teresita to looking over at me numerous times throughout the evaluation with a questioning look in his eye, seeming to say, *Is he for real?* (At least that's how I interpreted the look, as many of Dr. Dumasse's questions were out in far left field.) It seemed to me, and I could only imagine what Joe was thinking, that Dr. Dumassé either did not know what he was doing or felt as though the Veteran was wasting his time. Dr. Dumasse's whole demeanor was extremely off-putting. At one point Joe chimed in during one of the doctor's pauses between questions, focused directly on the doctor he asked, "Am I wasting your time? Because I feel as though you are looking at me and thinking I am wasting your time. I am here to get my knee checked out. I really do not need a lecture from you as far as not coming into the clinic earlier to be seen. If I am wasting your time, I will leave right now."

"Uh,... uh no,... ha, ha, ha... we're just um... trying to uh... figure out the best way to treat this," Dr. Dumassé finally choked out.

(I thought to myself – luckily, I hadn't spouted out what I had been thinking – ummm... *Find out what's wrong with his knee! Duh!*)

Ultimately, Dr. Dumassé decided not to do anything for the Veteran except give him Motrin and send him on his way. (No x-rays were ordered, follow-up scheduled with an orthopedist, or at the very least, a primary care provider appointment, or even physical therapy arranged, as Joe's pain was a worsening, albeit an ongoing, issue.)

Dr. Dumassé and Teresita then walked out and I sat in the room for a minute, closed my eyes and took a deep breath. Frankly, I was embarrassed. Joe came in for some sort of definitive treatment, or even a step in the right direction, to figure out what was going on with his knee. At the very least, we should have gotten current x-rays as it has been several *years* since he had had x-rays of his knee, and updated films would have been the prudent way to go, prior to obtaining a CT or MRI, should either of those become necessary. None of those concepts were suggested. Only Motrin.)

G.I. Joe then looked at me and said, "Does he know that he's dealing with trained killers?"

Slowly opening my eyes to his statement, I kind of chuckled to myself, knowing full-well that question was completely true. However, I've never really thought about that fact, only that we were there to treat fellow Veterans. That was definitely an interesting perspective.

Furthermore, his statement was certainly not a threat, just a Veteran frustrated with civilians attempting to treat them, with little or no respect or even understanding of their specific illnesses or injuries. In fact, other than job skills, when it came to medical issues, Veterans were not so different than civilians (yes, both groups have their whiners but, Veterans **on the whole** are more stoic). The goal was to figure out the problem and solve it, not continue to place a bandage over it and leave it to fester.

"I apologize. I realize that. . .," gesturing to Dr. Dumassé whom had just left, "was totally uncalled for."

"It's not your fault; he just doesn't need to come in here acting like he's above everyone else."

"I totally agree."

"Well hey, I thank you for your help, but I am going to go to my primary doctor out in town on my next day off and see if they can't take care of my knee."

"Again, I apologize, but remember what I said," referring to getting an x-ray and MRI or CT and getting it taken care of, "if you have the time, **please** let the patient rep know about this interaction. Nothing will get done if there's no paper trail of issues."

"I'll think about it."

Nodding, "That's all I can ask. Take care of yourself. And thank you for your service."

That whole incident happened before I realized who Dr. Dumassé truly was, a provider that was kicked out of numerous states for various unethical practices. He, as well as several others at the facility, undoubtedly, would never be able to attain a job in any other medical facility. Speaking mainly of civilian facilities. Therefore, they would always be the ones, from the bottom of the barrel, left to treat Veterans, and getting compensated quite well to do just that.

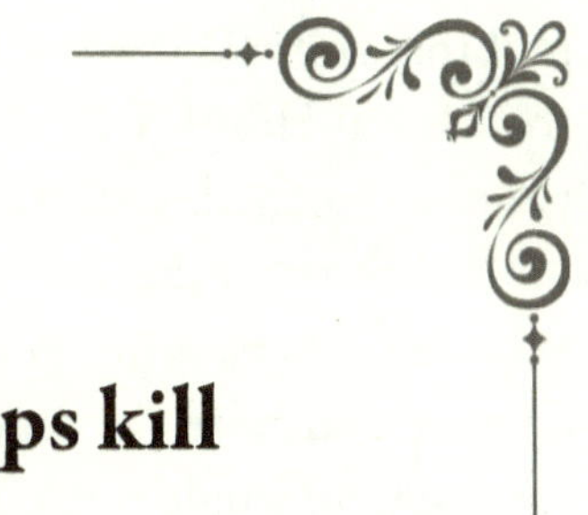

I'd rather the cops kill me...

On the *rare* occasion when the Mental Health department requested our assistance in medically clearing a Veteran for psychiatric admission or detox treatment, the staff would typically have their patients show up to our clinic in the middle to late afternoon. That would mean that by the time the lab results were completed and the Veteran was medically cleared, the Mental Health staff, most times, would no longer be found in the building in order to evaluate the Veteran. Therefore, we would be required to send them out to an appropriate facility, which would, on most occasions, take several hours to find transport, as we were in rural America and there are no real close facilities for detox or psychiatric treatment. Wait a minute... did I just say on the *rare* occasion that Mental Health required our assistance, where was my brain? I meant to say, on the habitual occurrence they required our assistance to clear ***their*** Veterans. It did not take me long to realize the *game* that the Mental Health providers were playing.

From the first day I started at the VA that had been an issue of *turfing (basically forcing their patients onto our clinic and therefore our responsibility)* their patients so that they would not have to complete the workups themselves. It became commonplace for the Mental Health department in the facility to do what they could so that their staff did not have to evaluate their own patients. Right! That's the way to care for our Nation's Veterans. (Yep, more sarcasm.) Mental Health was a big issue throughout the VA nationwide and this facility tried to pull that shit! Well, to be fair, the *higher-ups* in *management* allowed the Mental Health staff the ability to continuously get away with this practice. So, frankly, they are all to blame.

The fact that this custom bottle-necked our clinic was not really an issue, as far as *management* was concerned. Unless of course we racked up more and more overtime because of Mental Health's tactic, and then *management* would bitch, moan, and complain. There was no pleasing the *favorites,* whether that was a clinic or individual employee. (Once again, I digress.) We, the clinic staff, would do what we needed to do to get the Veterans the care they required. Although, as we seemed to be performing more and more of the Mental Health staff's duties, it allowed their staff the time to accomplish all of their other extra-curricular (oh, I mean collateral) duties as well as taking their required daily/hourly breaks. Referring back to those breaks spoken of previously, that we were very rarely afforded.

Our staff, for some insane reason, thought that continuing to argue with anyone in the role of *management* would ever get anything accomplished. At one point Dr. Lynn Fitzgerald, who was only with us for six to seven short months, finally got tired of being **dumped on** by other providers in the facility. She made it quite well known to whomever would listen, a hell-lotta good it ever did. Of course, being the competent provider that she was, she fully had our backing.

The whole issue came to a head one day shortly before my surgery and subsequent resignation. We had a Social Worker – Lim – (*SW – Significantly Worthless*) tell the mother of an adult Veteran, who lived a *close* two or three hours away, to bring her son into our clinic, to be evaluated and treated, and possibly admitted for suicidal thoughts. There were several issues with that situation:

1. Our clinic was over two to three hours away, and most likely another appropriate facility was closer and more appropriate to send the Veteran! Seriously, if the SW was that concerned to the patient's mental wellbeing and possible suicidal thoughts, Lim should have

directed them to the nearest emergency room, as any ***prudent*** provider would have done. (Sorry, where was my mind. I did say *prudent* provider, the definition of *prudent* meaning: "having or showing careful or good judgment". Regrettably, the providers I encountered definitely did not emulate *prudent* in that sense of the word.)

2. If the Veteran was decidedly actively suicidal, that was not simply a matter of the Veteran detoxing and needing medical clearance prior to outpatient treatment. That would be more of an issue for inpatient Mental Health treatment, meaning, being seen by a licensed MH provider.

Consequently, Lim, who was notorious for *evaluating* Veterans over the phone and/or sight unseen, told the Veteran's mother to bring her son into our clinic to be admitted for inpatient treatment! Then Lim actually wrote several notes in the Veteran's chart without even having laid eyes on or actually spoken with the patient. How in the world does that even happen? The reason I knew this was that the notes I read, written by Lim, had contradicted just about everything I had ascertained by evaluating the Veteran first-hand, actually visualizing and speaking with the Veteran, once he arrived. Definitely a concern for further investigation. In a perfect world that is, as that practice of writing up evaluations/assessments sight-unseen, in opinion, borders on malpractice. Not all *practicing* social workers in effect need to have a license, however it helps with attaining employment. Maybe that was the key, Lim was only *practicing*.

Back to the topic. Lim called our clinic around three-pm one Friday afternoon stating that he told the Veteran's mother to bring her son into us for detox and that they should be arriving around four-pm. Problem again was that they were at least two hours away. So it seemed as though Lim did not pass basic math in high school. (Had we been told that the Veteran was coming in for suicidal ideations, then Mental Health would've been required to stay and evaluate him. But the alleged complaint was for detox, and that was a *medical* issue which took precedence over mental health.)

Conveniently as was usual, the Mental Health staff would most definitely be out of the building by the time the Veteran even arrived, let alone being ready for evaluation. Knowing that the Veteran was on his way did not denote that they were required to remain in the building awaiting his arrival, to evaluate and treat **their own** patient. However, knowing they told the Veteran to report to our clinic, a *prudent* and even conscientious provider in that specialty should have waited around for their patient to arrive so that they could properly evaluate them. To reiterate, the definition of *prudent* allegedly was not applicable in this case.

AS WE WAITED FOR THE Veteran to arrive, I perused his electronic chart to check out his medical and mental health history to see what all we should expect. Lo and behold, there was a history and physical, written by Lim that same day. Weirdly enough, I wondered how that was possible as Lim never once saw, let alone spoke to, the Veteran that day to perform a proper history and physical. I received confirmation of Lim's (as we say in the Navy) *gun-decking*, (which basically means falsifying information or performing shoddy work) when I had the opportunity to speak with this Veteran in person. That was when I realized Lim had written false information in the Veteran's chart. That information could've be detrimental for the Veteran. How many other times had Lim performed that very same task?

When the Veteran did finally arrive in the clinic, I asked him straight up (yep, stuck again in triage as the first line of defense so to say), "What's going on today? Do you want to hurt or kill yourself?" His mom sat in the triage room with him, trying to tell me what she wanted me to know. Problem for her was, I wanted to hear from her twenty-something year-old son, what his thoughts were.

"No. I told my mom that I wanted help. After I got out of the military I got mixed up with drugs really bad and now I want to get off of them and get out of that whole scene. It got to the point that I made the statement, which my mom overheard, that if there were a drug bust that I was involved in and the cops showed up, I'd do what I had to do to have the cops kill me, because if I were ever caught, I'd rather have them shoot and kill me than to go back to prison."

Hmmm... made sense to me. Especially if he'd been in prison in the past, he knew what was in store for him and I supposed he had no desire to repeat the visit. Luckily enough I have never been in prison (as an inmate, that is). And, I have no freaking desire to experience that way of life. His explanation did not sound suicidal at all. Unless the thought of death over prison was considered a suicidal thought. If that were the case, then I am sure there are *a lot* of people out there that would be considered suicidal.

"When was the last time you used drugs?"

"It's been over three weeks now."

"Okay. Well, we got a call from Lim, a social worker from the Mental Health department, stating that you were coming in to detox and we need to medically clear you. That means that we need to check your labs and make sure there is no alcohol or drugs in your system. We'll need to do this before we can send you for inpatient treatment," I explained.

"What? I haven't used in over 3 weeks! This is insane! Isn't there anyway I can do outpatient treatment? I need to work and I don't want to lose my job. I don't want to go to prison, but I also don't want to lose the only job I have right now, " he remarked becoming slightly irritated, seeming almost homicidal. Not towards me, mind you, but towards this unseen entity in Mental Health. That super *prudent* social worker, Lim, who apparently could evaluate a patient without ever leaving his office *and* without ever having to see or even talk to the patient.

"Listen, let's get you taken care of now and worry about a job afterwards. Here is the contact information I have for another Veteran who hires only Veterans based on their specific skillset. Once you get out of the treatment facility, give him a call and see if he can help you." I wrote the contact information down for another Veteran that had just so happened to be in our clinic earlier that week explaining his company and asked that we pass on his information to any Veterans in need.

It didn't help that the Veteran's mother was not supportive of her late-twenty-something son, and basically forcing him to receive inpatient treatment. I guess that was one way to get older kids out of the house. How supportive!

Well, as was par for the course in our clinic, the *dumping* continued and the Veteran received the best care we could offer. He was medically cleared for transfer, and funny thing was... he had absolutely no drugs or alcohol whatsoever in his system. **Shocking**! We gave him some resources so that he could facilitate his admittance to our drug and alcohol rehab center once he was discharged from inpatient treatment. Yeah, interestingly enough, he wasn't admitted for suicidal ideations, which was practically unheard of for some odd reason. He was admitted for treatment of alcohol and drug use/abuse and detox of...??? Not really sure as he was not intoxicated or withdrawing. However, the turf to us and subsequently to the inpatient facility relieved all responsibility for treatment from the VA's mental health department.

NOT SURPRISING, WE learned several days later that the Veteran left the facility on his own accord. Unfortunately, he was not properly treated at all for the therapy that he had been initially seeking. But then again, Mental Health did not have to shoulder the burden of having to treat him either. Chalk one more up for them not having to treat their own patients. That's **all** that seemed to have mattered, that they (the

VA clinic) took care of their favorite employees. (Once again, blatant sarcasm. Ha!)

Sadly, I believe that Veteran went back to the life he was living prior to the entire Mental Health debacle. Maybe he had given a call to a company he was referred to that hired only Veterans based on their particular skills and specialty. If hired, he would have had to relocate, but he mentioned that that was not at all an issue. Considering the *super support* he was getting from his mother, I could only imagine he'd be more than happy to GTFO (Get the Fuck Out) of his house. Furthermore, I would fully understand if that Veteran was never seen by another VA provider. I would not blame him one bit. This is also one reason we have Veterans that have never been seen by a VA provider.

MANY VETERANS ARE TYPICALLY quite skeptical of the care they might receive at a VA clinic or hospital, for obvious reasons. One of those Veterans is described in the next chapter as another Veteran needing mental health support. He had never been seen at a VA clinic in over twenty years, and then the way he was treated when he finally came into our clinic was not surprising. Of course that story also occurred on a Friday evening. Must've been a thing about Fridays and Mental Health. Similar to the full moon phenomenon talked about in the ERs, I guess. However, I do wish this particular Veteran the best and hope he is doing well.

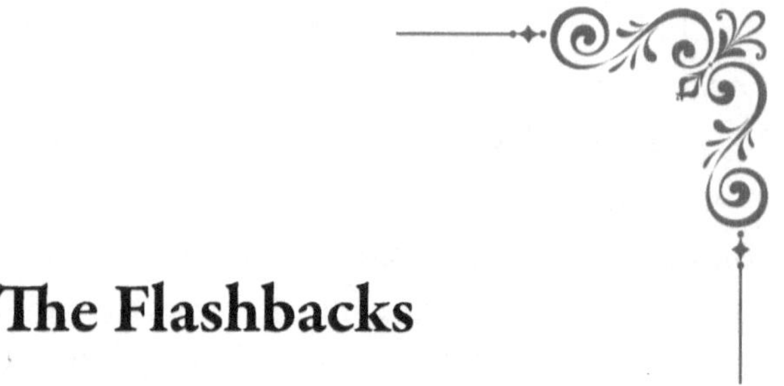

The Flashbacks

A Vietnam Era Veteran presented to the clinic late one Friday afternoon stating his buddy's nephew talked him into coming to the VA. This Veteran was one of the first Mental Health patients I had the pleasure of being introduced to during the first couple of months I was employed.

I am not sure what it was about Friday afternoons, but that seemed to be when everyone decided it would be a good time to be seen. Could it have maybe been avoidance therapy, (avoiding their issues and hoping they'd go away?) Or, maybe it was because they pondered the issue all week and then decided at the end of the week that they should probably be seen before the weekend?

Nevertheless, the Veteran apparently had been reluctant in the past because he had heard all sorts of horror stories about the VA and didn't want to be one more *casualty*, as well as he didn't want to die in a VA Medical Center. On arrival he proceeded to tell me that after speaking with his buddy's nephew and talking war stories (evidently his buddy's nephew had recently separated from the military), that was when he said the flashbacks started becoming too unbearable to handle on his own. He stated that almost every morning he'd wake up in a cold sweat after having a nightmare or flashback of his time overseas. He also informed me that his wife just did not understand and wanted to know why he was so angry and depressed all the time.

While talking with him, I guided him into one of our rooms and barely had time to sit him down in the chair before he all but lost it. He started tearing up, and his voice began to quiver when he spoke. But under the circumstances, he truly handled himself quite well. I asked him what we could do for him and that was when the dam broke and the waterworks commenced.

I don't pretend to be much of a *touchy-feely* type of nurse, and that was one reason I choose Emergency Nursing. Still, the gentleman was a fellow Vet. I couldn't help but feel some empathy and compassion for him as he was able to slowly get his thoughts out, albeit in pieces. Thoughts that had been, by all accounts, weighing on him for over twenty years. From what I could ascertain, he was in the military during the Vietnam War and had been held hostage in some underground bunker or Eastern European prison. He had frequent flashbacks of a foreign soldier holding a gun to his head threatening to pull the trigger while he laid face down on the filthy floor of his prison cell. He said he was tortured and his life threatened on numerous occasions. I had no desire to bring up those memories for him, but yes, a part of me wanted to know all of the *gory details*. Considering he was sitting there with me at that time, he made it through, physically unscathed anyway. Umm, yeah, what does one do? I politely excused myself when he was finished talking, knowing I was **way** out of my element. My morbid curiosity in wanting to know all of the details was in **no way** going to help the Veteran, and that was when I called in the *experts* from Mental Health.

As an acute care nurse, I was not extremely well equipped to handle that type of mental health issue, professionally at least. Although, I have had my fair share of *bizarre* patients, over the years, as well as those that were truly depressed and even psychotic. I'm much better able to handle the acute psychotic patient that is hyped up on drugs or alcohol, one that has overdosed on drugs, or even a patient that has had a mental lapse because of a simple lack of chemicals (not taking their medication). But, a patient, a Veteran, with significant Post Traumatic Stress Disorder (PTSD) was way out of my league. However, I learned from experience at the VA that my skills and experience were not as lacking as I thought, compared to the skills I'd seen in the Mental Health department.

Furthermore, being new to the VA myself, I was not all that accustomed with the functioning (or rather dysfunction) of that particular Mental Health department. Anywhere else I had worked, if we had a mental health patient, we would clear them medically, (make sure there was no medical reason behind the patient's symptoms such as drugs or alcohol, or even an electrolyte imbalance) and then contact a Mental Health specialist to evaluate and treat as they saw fit.

I'll admit, the VA was extremely eye-opening for me as that was so not the case there. The Mental Health department staff would rarely evaluate Veterans during normal working hours. To assess a Veteran towards the end of the day or week, and *after* hours was totally unheard of. As this particular Veteran was new to the system as well as the fact that he came in around 3pm on a Friday afternoon, no one in the Mental Health department would come to the clinic to even talk with, let alone evaluate him, especially since most were probably gone for the weekend.

As stated before, there was at least one Mental Health *professional* who had the uncanny *skill* of being able to evaluate and treat a Veteran sight-unseen. Their *professional* recommendation was to have the Veteran come back to the clinic Monday morning and get enrolled to see a primary care provider and have the primary care provider determine *if* the Veteran even needed to see a Mental Health *professional.*

Are you fucking kidding me? That grated on my last nerve. Total and complete laziness and incompetence at its best. That poor Veteran had never come to a VA for reasons such as those, and that was how he was treated. It was no wonder he never wanted to ever come to a VA in the past. And, I'd be surprised if he even came back. What did I do? Yep, another incident report written that went into the *twilight* or circular file in our *boss's* office. So yes, that Veteran was clearly suicidal and majorly depressed, yet our Mental Health department **refused** to see him. When in fact, he was clear of any drugs and alcohol. So, my question was this; what the hell good is a Mental Health department that refuse to see Mental Health Veterans?

I realized, and will openly admit, that Mental Health is not my forte. In fact, on-going craziness is definitely comic relief for me. And, when in the mood, I have been known to play into the delusions of my patients. Therefore, I was so totally **not** the best candidate to deal with Mental Health issues. Nonetheless, I was able to determine that this Veteran was sliding downhill fast and needed to talk to someone who could further assist. I could listen, but providing more than a sympathetic ear was beyond my scope of skills.

Unfortunately, when I called up to the Mental Health department I was informed in no uncertain terms that they would not see the patient. Period! **Wwwhhhaaattt???** The *clerk* I spoke with (apparently all the providers had left early for the weekend) said, "Our providers don't have to see any patient that they do not want to see."

Yep, those were their exact words. **Huh**? I then asked, "I'd like a copy of that instruction specifying this, please."

"Oh, you're going to have to go through your chain of command," was the **clerk's** response.

Again, **Huh**? Those civilians thought they know *What the Fuck* they were talking about, but actually, they had no freaking clue. That was painfully obvious when they spouted out words or phrases such as that above, akin to a mental health patient completely disconnected from society. I pondered their response and figured they thought that if they used some *military lingo* that they'd look like they knew what they were talking about, when in fact it actually made them look even more ignorant. Actually, I suppose that last statement would be an insult to any mental health patient, by comparing them to this level of incompetence. At least mental health patients completely disconnected from society had a reason for their actions, whereas the mental health staff did not.

I digress. I realized there was no use arguing with *stupid* and knowing that there was no way to fix or cure it, I hung up the phone. I didn't even bother being polite about it. The one regret I had was that I didn't write down the clerk's name.

So, not only would the Mental Health providers **not** see a patient after hours as needed (or at the end of the day, usually nearing the weekend or a holiday), they also would **only** see patients that they **chose** to see!

Of course, I looked at the clock. Yep, once again, by that time it was after 4pm on a Friday afternoon. Of course, no one would even think of staying late to see a patient (except of course our clinic staff, as we really had no choice).

Once I got off the phone with Mental Health, (muttering to myself how useless, once again, they were) I went back into the room with the Veteran and allowed him to just talk. He repeated his story of being in Eastern Europe during or after the Vietnam War, and held at gunpoint in some basement bunker where he was kept for close to a month.

In the midst of a break, I asked someone else to once again try and find a Mental Health provider to see that patient. I went so far as to ask the admin clerk to call the on-call provider. The admin clerk said they would call, but informed me he knew the on-call social worker wouldn't come in. That continued to be an on-going issue for the VA, and no one seemed to be making those staff members accountable for their indiscretions, even after the whole nationwide debacle of non-treatment of Veterans in need of mental health assistance. The Mental Health staff at this VA appeared to act as though they were untouchable. Additionally, based on how upper *management* handled the issues with them, apparently, they **were** untouchable.

RETURNING TO THE MAIN concern, we finally managed to get the Veteran an appointment that following Monday with one of the Nurse Practitioners in the primary care clinic. Fortunately that particular NP was one of the few that was well respected **and** had extensive experience with mental health patients.

Furthermore, this Veteran, being new to the clinic, did not know where anything was or where to go. I walked him around a bit and showed him where he would need to go for his appointment that following Monday. I then informed him if he needed to see/talk to **anyone** before his appointment that he should call the triage nurse line (and I provided him the number) or to go to the nearest Emergency Room. He agreed and as I walked him out, I gave him a huge hug and told him we were there Monday through Friday if he ever needed us. I then sent up a quick prayer that he would get through the weekend without issues, and make it safely to his appointment that following Monday.

It was just amazing that Veterans were even able to be seen in the Mental Health clinic, the way the staff treated most of those Veterans. I had witnessed them do whatever they could to **not** see a patient, rather than take a few extra minutes and actually speak with and evaluate a Veteran. It was no wonder that Veteran even came into the clinic, as it seemed that some of the stories he had heard were in fact very true.

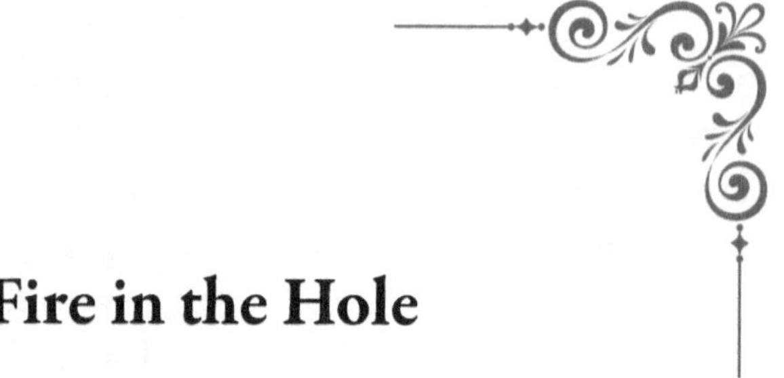

Fire in the Hole

So, there I was, sitting behind the nurse's station, charting on one of the many patients that had come in that day. I just so happened to be facing out towards the four rooms of the clinic when Gus, the *manager* of the outpatient clinic, rushed in, appearing frazzled. He looked as though he was unable to formulate a comprehensible sentence, even a short one. He was apparently out of breath. Maybe he should cut down on one of his six-plus smoke breaks a day and work out a little, or maybe just work, after all, he was younger than I was. Unfortunately, that was not saying much, however, still true.

Either way, seeing that Gus was gasping when he sagged against the counter, attempting to catch his breath, I went back to charting on one of my many previous patients. In the midst of typing, Gus finally gasped, and then spurted out rather excitedly, "There's a guy in the clinic who has a piece of hot metal stuck in his ear and he's going to need to be transferred out!" Once spilling that out, Gus kind-of just sagged on the nurse's station to catch his breath.

I was almost certain that I looked at him as though he was crazy. I thought to myself, *And you're telling ME this... why?* Then I thought there must be a reason he rushed over here as Gus never seemed to hurry anywhere. I peeked up at the clock on the wall behind where Gus chose to stand. (The staff in our clinic were not much of *clock watchers* as other employees in the VA seemed to be, for the simple fact that we were never really afforded the ability to actually leave work *on time*, whatever that was, or even early for that matter). The clock showed

4:15pm. I then glanced back at Gus, not saying a word. I immediately knew what the issue was, and I went about with my charting. It wasn't as though he couldn't transfer a patient out himself. The problem was, it would've taken longer than the 15-minutes he had left on his shift and Gus didn't seem to care if we would had to remain late... again. Wondering to myself, *What did you do for him?* I knew what the answer would be before it even left his mouth... nothing. But, being the glutton for punishment or just the sarcastic bitch that I am, out loud I had to ask, "What have you done for the patient?"

Of course Gus's response was no surprise at all. "Nothing! He has hot metal stuck in his ear." Then he repeated, "He needs to be sent out immediately!"

Well, get on it!

I knew it'd be useless for me to even ask if anyone actually looked to see if there was in fact a piece of metal stuck in the Veteran's ear. It would just be akin to poking the bear, just to satisfy my curiosity as to whether they were even competent enough to evaluate a true emergency. In fact, if it were a true emergency, why in the hell was Gus wasting time hurrying down the hall to our clinic only to inform us of the need to have the Veteran transferred out when all Gus needed to do was dial 9-1-1!!! ***Hello****....* Anyone with a brain could've figured that out. In fact, it was common knowledge, or so I thought, in the clinic to do just that. Guess I was mistaken, once again.

"So, send him out," I stated bluntly, not wanting to spend more time on his theatrics than necessary. "You can send him out from the clinic, just as easily as we can here. If it's a true emergency, all you need to do is dial 9-1-1," I said somewhat frustrated that he chose to bother me with a trivial matter that he should've solved by one simple phone call. There I went, with common sense.

My comment was met with... silence. Gus once again repeated, "He has hot metal stuck in his ear."

I must've liked poking the bear. Maybe that was my comic relief. With an irritated sigh I slowly lifted my head up from focusing on the computer I had been charting on and eyed Gus stating, "And you are wasting time over here when the ambulance could have already picked him up and taken him to the ER. If it is truly an emergency."

Oh, he didn't seem to like that one bit. He was a *manager*, and us *peons* just don't talk to *management* as the idiots they truly were. So, once again I got delivered a look as though he'd like to shoot me dead right then and there, or at the very least take me out back and try like hell to kick my ass. Okay, I'll bite. After Gus didn't respond to my statement I continued with, "What have you all done for him?"

"The nurse triaged him and told me what she found. I suggested we bring him over here, knowing he'll need to be transferred out."

There were still *sooooo* many problems with that statement. First of all, like I said, if it truly was an emergency, the clinic staff, should have just called 9-1-1. Or, if they thought we could evaluate and treat him and maybe then transfer him out if needed, they would've called over instead of wasting his time running down the hall to our clinic. Better yet, do what they normally do and just bring him over without any **heads up** at all, and *dump* the patient on us.

I continued poking the bear. "Just so am I understanding this correctly, you have not yet done anything for him?"

"No, he needs to be transferred out immediately!"

My very next thought was, then how in the hell Gus knew the Veteran needed to be transferred out if the nurse hadn't even done anything for the patient. Furthermore, they were wasting time if it truly was an emergency!

"If that's the case, then call 911," I reiterated matter-of-factly. (Duh! **Oh My God**, I was surrounded by idiots.) I looked back at Dr. Lynn right then and she wouldn't even look my way. I knew she was listening to our entire interaction and she just kept shaking her head and chuckling to herself.

Knowing that Gus was several beers short of a six-pack I conceded, "Well, then bring him over now. I don't want to be here all night, either," I said tersely. I then continued with, "And in the future, if you have a patient that has a true emergency, call 9-1-1 like we are all supposed to do in the event of a true emergency," I instructed, and went back to my charting. I completely ignored Gus after that.

Knowing I was not going to give him another thought or any additional attention, as he was used to being the center of attention, he then left to go get the Veteran, finally.

THE VETERAN WAS ESCORTED over to our clinic within a few minutes. I met him at the door and walked with him into a room. I allowed him time to sit down, saying "Sir, please have a seat". He was shaking his head the entire time and so I asked, after I shut the door to the room, and we were both sitting down, "What's going on? What happened?"

He responded with, "I was welding at work and a drop of hot metal flew up into my ear. (Now mind you I actually let him continue telling his story rather than interrupt him, stop him right there and freak out like the clinic nurse apparently did.) I flushed it with water and it's still burning."

And there it was! The clinic nurses were just so ***special.*** (That may be interpreted anyway in which seems to fit.) Without even needing a patient to finish their explanations/story, those nurses apparently ***knew*** what was going on even more so than the Veteran did. Not!!!

I couldn't help but start to laugh out loud. Finally catching my breath I stated, "Sir, I apologize, but I am still trying to figure out why the other nurses felt as though you needed to be rushed over here and transferred out immediately. Didn't you tell them the same thing you just told me?"

"I started to; however they would not allow me to finish my story."

Shocking!!! It wasn't as though his story was ***super*** long.

"Has anyone even looked in your ear since you got here?"

"Not yet." *Of course not.*

"Alrightly then. Is it okay if I take a look in your ear?"

"Finally!" He exclaimed. "Sounds good to me," he added, sounding relieved.

The *young* man (probably well into his sixties) was extremely calm, polite and just wanted someone to listen to his concerns and take care of his immediate medical needs.

I used the otoscope and looked in his good ear first and then the ear that had been affected, next. I could not visualize any foreign body in either ear. "Sir, I don't see anything in your ear. All I can tell is that it's red and appears irritated. Of course, I'm just the nurse. I will have the doctor verify my findings in a bit. You said no one looked in your ear in the clinic before they rushed you over here, correct?"

"No, like I said, they didn't even let me finish telling them that I flushed my ear with water."

"As you should have. My apologies, I didn't mean to cut you off."

"No problem. Like I said, I flushed it out immediately. I've done this before," he added sheepishly.

At that I gave him what I could only image to be a goofy questioning look.

"I know, I should be more careful," he stated somewhat embarrassed, smiling, which made me also smile.

"But you flushed it out and probably washed out the metal that was in there. That's probably all we would've done for you. Any problems with your hearing?"

"Nope, not at all."

"Okay, well let me go speak with my doctor and I do not see any reason we would need to transfer you out to an ***Emergency Room***," I said chuckling at the absurdity. "We'll probably give you some drops for your ear to help with the pain and to prevent an infection. I'll be back in a little bit after I've spoken with the doctor."

He nodded his head and thanked me.

Walking to the nurse's station and over to where Dr. Fitzgerald was sitting, she looked at me like *I want to hear this extremely emergent scenario and maybe I'll believe that the clinic nurses are actually competent at their job*, not! I started with, "Hey doc, this is the guy from the clinic. He was welding and a drop of hot metal flew up and got stuck in his ear. Immediately afterwards he flushed out his ear. The ear canal is red and appears irritated, but I don't see any metal or other foreign bodies in his ear. He is not having any problems hearing and says this has happened in the past at which time he flushed the ear out copiously and did the same today. I personally do not see any need for us to necessitate transferring him anywhere (I said laughingly as I couldn't seem to help myself). I have no idea why the clinic could not have handled this patient themselves, other than it is the end of the day... again. Those nurses have no idea how to do competent patient care, let alone triage. First and foremost they would need to listen. That is apparently is a huge undertaking for them as had they actually listened to him, they would've heard that he flushed out the ear, and done what I am doing right now, talk to the doctor. Then have the doctor take a look, write him a prescription for ear drops - analgesic and possibly antibiotic and send him on his way." Catching my breath I added, "Sorry, I am rambling and just venting my frustration at the stupidity of it all. Once again, the clinic has dumped yet another patient on us."

The look Dr. Fitzgerald gave me then was one of complete understanding and solidarity. However, she didn't say anything to be overheard by the patient. Adding, "Okay, let him know I'll be in a couple of minutes."

I walked back into the room and informed the Veteran that the doctor would be in shortly, very shortly as she seemed to follow me into the room and was then standing right behind me. (Quick and sneaky/stealthy was Dr. Lynn.) The Veteran then proceeded to tell her the same story he had just told me, and as a good prudent medical professional, she of course actually listened to him. She then took a look in his ear, seeing the same thing I did, nothing other than redness.

"Well sir, looks like my nurse here is right. There's no need to transfer you out. I'll write you a prescription for some ear drops and we'll get you out of here. Do you have any questions?"

"No ma'am, I'm good. Thank you."

It took Dr. Lynn maybe 10-15 minutes to finish up the patient's chart and order the medications for him. As I got ready to discharge him, I glanced up at the clock and noted it was only 5pm. Hmmm, interesting, how the clinic staff did not want to spend one more minute on the gentleman as they might've had to stay an extra half an hour later than their usual quitting time. (Or rather, what we *assumed* was their usual quitting time. For all we knew, their normal quitting time was maybe hours prior).

AS I PREPARED TO OFFER the Veteran his discharge papers and information, I also informed him that the pharmacy would be open while we still had patients and he was free to go down there at that time and pick up his medications. I also told him I had called ahead to activate those prescriptions and that they should be ready for him by the time he got there. Unless he had any further questions, he was free to go. Once he signed his discharge papers, he was out of the clinic in a flash. Again, we did what we could to care for our Veterans, even the ones that no one else seemed to want to be bothered with.

Lights Out

The time was sixteen-forty-five on a, yep surprise, Friday afternoon (4:45pm for civilian folks – or anyone unfamiliar with the twenty-four-hour clock – as we used to say frequently in the military) and we were almost out (*early*) for the weekend. That would've been the first time in who knew how long. I checked with the admin clerk to see if we missed anyone, and prayed that no one else came in before five, so that we could actually get out of work on time, for once. At the admin desk I noticed a lone man sitting in the waiting room and looked quizzically at, Dave.

It was then when he finally decided to pipe up, "I know this Veteran is empaneled (assigned) to one of the clinics in the building. However, he has been sitting in the clinic waiting area to be seen for the last three hours. He came in around lunchtime and was told he would be seen in between patients as a walk-in. All he needed was to get his medication refilled. Can we help him out?"

"Um, come again? What kind of medication is he wanting refilled?" I figured I had heard Dave all wrong seeing as a medication refill should've been a quick visit for the clinic staff. Unless of course it was for narcotics, and then that might've taken a little longer. However, a simple medication refill should've taken five, or maybe ten minutes out of their day. That should have been a simple enough task for his primary care nurse to accomplish relatively effortlessly, and then send him on his way within a few minutes. Oh wait, that would've been five or ten minutes out of their many breaks during the day. Whatever was I thinking?

Dave basically repeated what he had just told me, continuing with, "He came up to me a little while ago saying he was sitting in the waiting room over there (meaning the primary care clinic waiting room) and they started turning off all the lights and left him sitting there in the dark. No one asked him what he was doing there or if he needed assistance. All he wanted was his blood pressure medication refilled cause he doesn't have enough to get him through the weekend."

I took a deep breath, counted to five in my head (because I was too pissed to count all the way to ten).

One...

Two...

Three...

Four...

Five...

Pause...

Then, "You've got to be fucking kidding me!"

Pause...

I continued with, "You're not kidding... and I am not one bit surprised."

Taking a deep, cleansing breath, I then turned and walked over to the Veteran sitting in our waiting room, and thankfully out of earshot of my last bout of *Lacking a Filter*.

Smiling I began with, "Good afternoon, sir. Would you like to follow me back to see what all we can do for you?" I escorted him back to the triage area. "How are you doing this evening? " Before he could even answer I continued with, "I am sorry that you had to wait so long to be seen. What can I do for you?"

"I just need this medicine refilled," he started, showing me the empty bottle. He continued, "I went over there around noon today because I knew I did not have enough to make it through the weekend to get it refilled on Monday."

"That's all you need?" I asked in astonishment. (All the while shaking my head.) "We can certainly help you out. Do me a favor, sit right there, I'll go speak to our doctor. We are not extremely busy right now, and as it's Friday afternoon everyone's getting ready to head out shortly. However, I think I can get them to write you a refill for a month, or at the very least enough to last you through until you can get back in to see your Primary Care Provider next week."

"That would be wonderful. Thank you," stated the quiet old man, who couldn't be much younger than eighty.

I walked to the back of the clinic and spoke with Dr. Fitzgerald, explaining the situation. She then looked at me like she was literally dumbfounded and shocked that something like that would *ever* happen here at the VA.

"Really? Are you surprised in the least?...(*Pause*) Seriously?" I asked.

Shaking her head, she muttered, "Of course not. This is par for this place." Meanwhile, she took a minute out of her busy schedule, finishing up for the day, to input the prescription refill for the gentleman. What a horrible burden, I tell you (oops, a little sarcasm).

I returned to the triage room where I had left the elderly Veteran and informed him that our doctor had ordered the medication for him. He should have enough to last through the next month, so that he would have time to see his primary care provider before he would need another refill. I then called the pharmacy, explained the situation to the tech, and asked them to start processing the medication so that the *young* man, who had waited all day for a simple refill, could get home. He had about an hour's drive, and it was starting to get dark. I was appalled that he had been at the clinic for over four or five hours that day waiting for a uncomplicated refill.

AFTER I WALKED THE Veteran out of the triage room and directed him down the hall towards the pharmacy, I went back to the triage desk to write up my note. Once finished, I left the triage room and went back to the admin clerk's desk to check and see if there were any *other* Veterans that were left by the clinic staff or anyone else needing to be seen before the weekend.

No more Veterans were around; however I did see the clinic nurses walking down the hallway at that time, from their clinic, leaving for the weekend. Somehow I knew they were the clinic nurses for our last Veteran. I stopped them along their route and asked what had happened, as one of their patients was left in the waiting room and the lights had been turned out on him. It was apparent that no one had checked the waiting room before getting ready to leave for the evening, and for the weekend. I also informed them that he had walked-in needing a refill of his blood pressure medicine.

"Oh, he can come back Monday," the RN or LVN stated with a dismissive wave of her hand. Unfortunately for her, she did not seem to know that I was not one to buy into her very rude and insensitive response uttered with a haughty attitude.

"No. He can't!" I practically yelled. Ooooh how I wanted to throttle them both for even thinking that. "He drove an hour to get here. He patiently waited over three hours because he was told **he would be seen** as a walk-in to get his medications refilled. The PACT nurse told our triage nurse that he would be seen. But, he was left sitting in the waiting room while the lights were all turned out and you all were getting ready to leave for the weekend. You left him sitting there in the dark, in the waiting room while everyone packed up to go home for the weekend. Everyone seemed to conveniently ignore the fact that he was still sitting there, waiting for his medication to be refilled. He sat there for over **three hours** because he was *told* by a clinic nurse that it would get done by the end of the day. Sorry, wrong answer!"

They both just looked at me, shrugged their shoulders, and one then stated, "Well, you took care of him then, right? Then there's no problem," again with the laissez-faire, haughty attitude.

Lucky for them I had a lot of experience with patience in the military. *Hurry up and wait* was a common mantra. Once more, I took a deep, somewhat cleansing breath and yet again opened my mouth. (Yeah, I know I was not so good about using filters most of the time, but I tried, sort-of). "Yes, there most certainly *is* a problem. You all don't seem to get the fact that you guys, in essence abandoned a Veteran. You left an eighty-year-old Veteran sitting in the waiting room while you shut out all the lights, completely ignoring the fact that there was someone still waiting to be seen. You just blew off someone who had a very simple request; *and* was told he would be taken care of *today*! I *will* be writing this up. This is completely unsat (unsatisfactory)"

Again, those two nurses looked at each other, rolled their eyes and walked off as though the incident was not a big deal. Luckily I had known their names with which to add to my write-up.

That was yet another write-up that would most likely go unacknowledged by the *higher-ups*, and those two nurses seemed to know that, simply by their reaction to my statement about being written up. Unfortunately, there was not enough accountability or responsibility accepted by many of the employees, especially the nurses, from what I had observed. Quite sad in fact, considering it was the Veterans that suffered when staff members such as those were enabled, by *management*, to continue their lack of treatment without incorporating the VA's core values of 'i. c.a.r.e.' (Integrity, Commitment, Advocacy, Respect, Excellence).

Those two nurses violated all five values *and* ultimately were not held accountable by their *supervisor*. Nevertheless, I figured, if I inundated Bertha's email, as well as her *boss's*, with observed occurrences of neglect and/or abandonment of Veterans, then I was doing the best job that I could in a situation of incompetent *leadership*. Unfortunately, it still did not sit well with me that nothing seemed to ever be done in cases such as those. In fact, even the Inspector General didn't seem to care about concerns with regards to patient neglect or abandonment, unless maybe a patient were to die, and I was not willing to let that happen. As is turned out, shoddy nursing seemed to elicit a promotion for the responsible nurses and supervisors of those nurses.

Okay, the soap-box tirade is over, for now. We were, fortunately, able to get the gentleman's prescription refill ordered and he was sent to the pharmacy to pick up the medications and then sent on his way home, an hour away, but that had not always been the case.

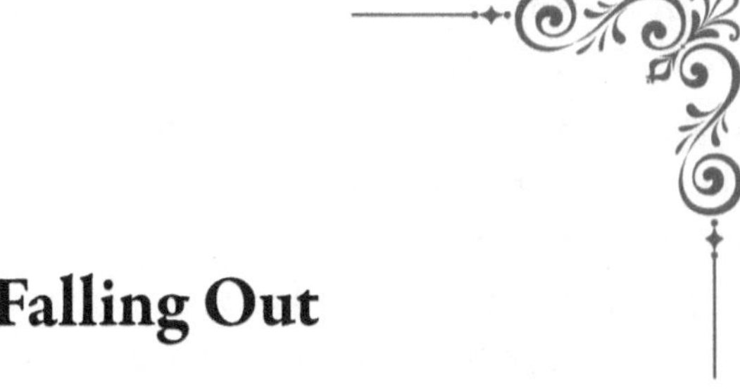

Falling Out

One evening around 6pm we were *surprisingly* still taking care of patients (oops, more sarcasm). At that time the rest of the facility staff had been gone for over an hour or two and we had stopped checking in patients close to an hour prior. However, we still had patients that needed to be treated and dispositioned. That was when the admin clerk came to the back of the clinic and asked, "So, what are we going to do with this guy out here in the waiting room?"

Quizzically, I looked at him like *What the Fuck are you talking about? It's 6 o'clock.* So I asked, "Did you seriously just check someone else in?"

"You know I wouldn't do that, but I told Markus about this guy, (who was the triage nurse that day) and I am waiting to find out what to do with him."

"Who is it? Where did he come from? What does he need?" I rapidly tossed questions his way.

"The clinic nurse walked him over here to the waiting room a little while ago, and then told me she couldn't wait with him any longer as she had to go home and left him sitting there in the waiting room. He doesn't look all that good. You might wanna come check on him."

"*WHAT*?" I practically yelled. "The clinic nurse dumped a patient in our waiting room and didn't bother to let any of us know that the patient was even out there? What's wrong with him?" But, before I got too worked up I did ask around to my fellow co-workers, "did any of you accept a patient from the clinic?"

A resounding "no, uh-no," went through my co-workers in the clinic. Then I thought to ask the provider, a Nurse Practitioner, not that they wouldn't have told us, but it might've been last minute and they got caught up in doing something else and simply just forgot to mention it. Their answer was pretty much the same,... sort-of. Their response was, "there's another Veteran that we haven't checked in yet?"

"Let me go find out what is going on." At that, I followed the admin clerk (Dave) back out to the waiting room, asking as we went, "What's going on with him?"

"He just doesn't look good," was the answer I received.

At that, I was sure I mumbled something under my breath, like, *"and the nurse **just left him** out there in the waiting room???"*

Arriving in the waiting room, we found a very sleepy looking elderly Veteran, sitting by himself in a chair at the end of the room.

I walked up to him and started with, "Hi sir. How are you doing tonight? How are you feeling?"

He glanced at me with a somewhat dazed look, as though he was trying to focus, and mumbled something that neither I nor Dave could understand.

"Sir, what's your name?"

He was able to supply us his name without too much difficulty.

"Sir, what year is it?"

He mumbled the year correctly.

Okay, we were doing okay thus far. Still, there was just something *off* about him.

"Sir, what brought you into the clinic today?"

"My blood pressure was high," he answered rather clearly.

"Okay, what did the doctor do for your blood pressure?"

"Um, I think they gave me some medicine," he muttered.

"How are you feeling right now?"

Instead of answering, he stumbled out of the chair, turned the corner and headed over to the water fountain. Dave and I just kind of glanced at each other, not taking our eyes off of the gentleman. After getting himself a drink from the water fountain, he stumbled back towards us and we both sort-of caught him before he did a faceplant right there on the hard tile floor. One of us was on either side of him and walked/carried him towards the back of the clinic and proceeded to get him settled in the first available room.

Once we got him released onto the gurney I checked his vital signs. I obtained a blood pressure reading of 70/30. Yeah, that was just a little too low for my comfort, considering I had absolutely no idea what was going on with the gentleman. I then asked Leslie to obtain an EKG and meanwhile I grabbed an IV start kit, all the while telling Dave to call 911. After grabbing the IV start kit and a bag of fluid, I informed the Nurse Practitioner that we would be sending the Veteran out.

The nurse practitioner used that time to say, "We can order some labs, get an x-ray and..."

Putting my hand up, I cut him off and didn't let him continue on that train of thought. I politely, but firmly informed the Nurse Practitioner, "We are calling 911. I have no idea why his blood pressure is so low, and we have no capabilities here to take care of him if he's having a stroke, a heart attack, a ruptured aneurysm, or any other number of issues. We're calling 911!"

He again tried to get us to order labs and x-ray and maybe a CT, of which none of those staff members were currently present in the building as everyone had left for the evening. We would've had to call a representative back from each of those departments, and who knew how long that'd take.

"We have time to do an EKG and maybe insert an IV to get fluids infusing before EMS arrives. That's all we're doing. We are not going to sit around and delay his care by waiting for an x-ray tech to respond to a page or labs that we will not be able to do much about if they are grossly abnormal. It's after six o'clock and all of the ancillary services are gone for the day," I kindly but firmly put my foot down on the issue.

The Nurse Practitioner turned back around and went back to charting or whatever he had been doing when we brought the patient in. I contacted the local ER and spoke to the nurse, giving them a brief report, just as EMS personnel arrived.

AFTER EMS LEFT WITH the patient in tow I got to thinking about earlier in the day when one of the clinic nurses was having a hard time accessing the Pyxis machine in the med room. When I let them into the room, they withdrew a second dose of 0.2mg of Clonidine, a potent blood pressure medicine, for that very same patient. At the time, when the patient was in our gurney, I was not aware that it had been that very same patient. As I looked back on that moment and thought to myself, as an ER nurse I've rarely given a total of 0.2mg of Clonidine let alone *two* doses, within one hour, to the same patient. I do remember asking the nurse if they were sure they wanted to give that amount.

That nurse at the time had responded with, "That's what the doctor ordered." I remember shaking my head, and decided it was none of my business. I probably should've stepped in (most-likely overstepping my responsibilities, as the patient was not our responsibility) and done a little more investigating.

I then asked the nurse how high the patient's blood pressure was and if it was high enough that he needed a massive dose such as that, maybe he should be in our clinic where we could've kept a better eye on him, including monitors which were few and far between (if at all) in the clinics. After all, the clinic urgently sent over patients with bunions, but the Veterans that *really* needed to be in an acute clinic rarely were. It made no sense. Frankly, it was almost as though they'd rather kill them in the clinic then have us save them. (Okay, so a little more sarcasm, based on a just a *smidgen* of truth.)

WITH THAT NEW INSIGHT, as it was shortly after EMS wheeled the patient out, I went into the med room and pulled up the patient's name on the Pyxis. Sure enough, both doses of the Clonidine had been for him. Well shit! No wonder his blood pressure was so freaking low. I then looked through his chart to see what his blood pressure was *prior* to being given such a high dose of the medication. It was only systolic in the 160's and diastolic like in the 90's. Oh My God! I rarely have given patients with that blood pressure *any* medication in the ER, let alone two hefty doses of Clonidine. If I were to give Clonidine, it would've been like an eighth to a quarter of the dose that was given. After fuming and sputtering about the insolence and ignorance of both the clinic provider and nurse for not doing their due diligence, I finally took a huge, calming breath. That was when I called the local ER and spoke with the same nurse I had just given report to and told them I knew why the patient's blood pressure was so low. When I told the nurse, they had the same reaction as I had. "They gave *how much clonidine*?"

"Yep, he got a total of 0.4mg of Clonidine in less than an hour timeframe." As ER nurses, we both knew that it could take over an hour for the medication to kick in and therefore, after reviewing the chart, I saw that he was given one dose, and then half an hour later was given another dose. His blood pressure was checked at the hour mark from the first dose of medication which was probably just starting to kick in then. In fact, the Veteran's initial blood pressure was nowhere near high enough to even warrant 0.2mg of an initial dose of the medicine. I would've started with 0.05 or 0.1mg, but hey, who was I but *just* the nurse, and obviously the *red-headed step-child* of the VA clinic nurses.

ONCE THAT WHOLE DEBACLE was finally over, I went out to the clerk and vented; not at him, but to him. "What happened? What was that veteran doing here in the first place?"

That was when Dave told me about the nurse from the clinic basically dumping the Veteran in the waiting room and then telling him that they couldn't stay with the Veteran anymore because they had to go home.

I asked him "Why the Fuck did they not come talk to one of us and do a proper hand-off if that was the case? That's considered patient abandonment and completely unethical. Seriously, I don't want to stay here any longer than *I have to* either, but because of their negligence, he could've had a lot worse happen to him by just abandoning him here in the waiting room. That's patient abandonment, pure and simple. This shit just pisses me off, and no one here seems to care one iota. I am going to write this one up, too, but unfortunately, we both know what that'll do, absolutely nothing! Nothing seems to ever happen when patients *almost* die. Oh wait, unless it's something we here in the clinic allegedly fuck up and then they sick a witch hunt on us. Kind of like they did to me about four months ago when I was not right next to a patient constantly, although he was never alone in this *huge*, five bed clinic. And, in fact, at one point that patient was even being watched by the Chief *nurse* for close to twenty minutes. So in reality, that was not a fuck-up on our part, but just a run-of-the-mill witch hunt. Probably for shits and giggles!" Okay, I think that was probably the end of my tirade for the evening.

LIKE IT'S BEEN SAID often, it's not *what* you know, but *who* you know, that gets one a job, a promotion, or even cleared from any wrong-doing like patient neglect or abandonment. Hence, with my big mouth and prior experience as an ER nurse, as well as a leader, I'd go nowhere in the VA system. I state this simply because I was not sleeping with the right people or person, as well as I was very outspoken about the mistreatment of Veterans that I had witnessed firsthand..

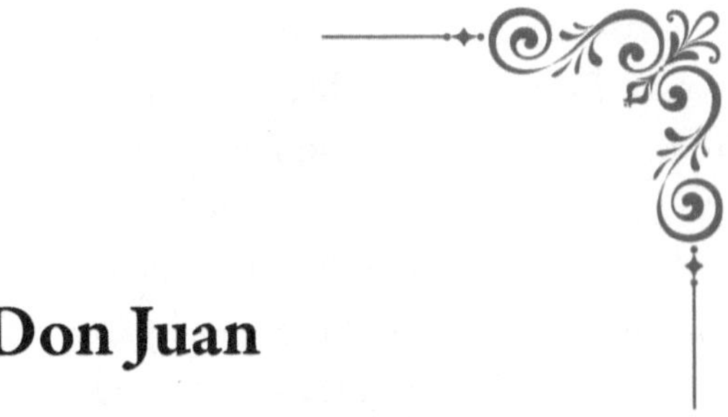

Don Juan

I t was the end of another very long day and I had made a point to check the waiting room, as I did most days prior to closing up and going home. I wanted to see if we had any other Veterans that may have slipped through the cracks and needed attention. I happened upon a LOM (little old man) sitting quietly on one of the double-seaters in the waiting room. As he was the only one left in the waiting room, I went up to him and asked, "Sir, do you mind if I sit here?" motioning to the empty space on the double seat next to him.

He looked at me, "Do I know you?" He asked quietly, meanwhile patting the seat next to him, assumingly my cue to sit down.

Taking his cue, I sat down next to him and turned to face him, eyeing his World War II ball cap he proudly displayed, and asked, "World War II, huh? What did you do?"

"I was a Navy Gunnersmate. Way before your time," he stated proudly.

"Well, thank you for your service and I am glad you made it home safely."

He seemed to brush off my gratitude, as so many Veterans tended to do when their service was mentioned and/or congratulated. (From experience it has seemed that most Veterans do not like to remember or even flaunt their service to our country) He then paused before stating, "You know, you look like someone I knew."

Pondering his statement, I had heard that more times than I could count. I don't know what it was about me but so many people seemed to know someone that looks like me. Must be my Polish nose. ☺

"Really, who might that be?"

"Oh, I am not really sure, but I'll tell you," pausing, he continued "you're married, right? I can see by that ring on your finger."

"Yes sir, that's right, I am married."

"Well, if you weren't married and I wasn't so old..." he drifted off.

"Well, how old are you?"

"Ninety-three," he stated incredibly proud. He sat more upright and puffed out his chest.

"Well, you are kind of cute," I started. "But yes, I am married and I love my husband very much and am very happy in fact."

"He's a very lucky man."

"Why thank you. I like to think so. Are you married?"

"Naw. I was a player in my time." He smiled as he mentioned that, sounding extremely proud of his skills with the ladies.

"What do you mean *was*? It seems to me that you are still very much the player. I mean, you're flirting with me right now, even knowing I am married," I stated jokingly and with a chuckle.

He outright laughed at that. "My time is up for that. I just try to make it through one day at a time these days."

"Well, you seem to be doing just fine for yourself. You remind me of my great uncle, also a World War II Vet who is your age, and just as ornery," I responded with a smile.

"But, not as good looking I'm sure," he countered.

Chuckling, "I'm going to have to tell him you said that."

Another brief pause and my Don Juan stated, "Well, I've taken up way too much of your time as it is. I should be on my way. My medicines should be ready soon."

"Not at all. It was a pleasure speaking with you. Are you sure that there is nothing we can do for you?"

"Oh heavens no. I am just going to pick up my medications and then I will be getting on home."

"Okay. I was just checking because I didn't want to leave you sitting here if you were waiting for us to see you."

I paused for a moment and then, double checking, asked, "So, you're sure there is nothing you need us to do for you?"

"I am quite sure. I am quite sure ma'am." (For the most part, Veterans are the most respectable people one will ever meet).

"Well sir, you have a good night, drive safe, and it was such a pleasure talking with you." I then just smiled at him, patted and shook his hand before I got up and walked back to the clinic. I turned only once to check on him and smile and wave. I was so ready to go home for the evening after a very long and busy day.

Days like that, busy as it was, I don't remember any of the other crap that ensued. I only recalled that I was lucky enough to be able to spend even a few minutes speaking with a World War II Vet, as there are so few left in this world. That in itself was the highlight of my day. ☺

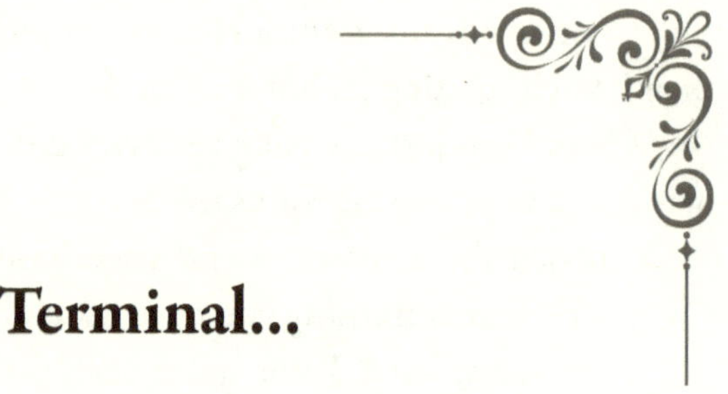

Terminal...

It seemed as though we might've seen at least one *interesting* or comical patient a day, rarely two or more. One of those days, a surprisingly older Veteran (just a little more sarcasm, not about the Veteran, just the fact that he was older, as many were) presented to the clinic requesting to have his pain medications refilled. As noted previously as well as with the laws specifying that narcotics could not be prescribed (or refilled) by anyone other than the patient's Primary Care Provider, in our clinic we were not allowed to prescribe or refill any narcotics for those Veterans that were on chronic pain meds. If a Veteran attempted to push the issue to get those medications filled by anyone other than their primary care provider, then they could possibly lose the ability to receive any narcotics all together through the VA system. This appeared to become a pattern throughout the VA system, and I have written several vignettes related to this topic.

Well, as was the way of the VA for *years*, it was an accepted practice for Veterans to become treated with (aka *hooked* on) narcotics for most ailments of the population. Funny that it was "Vitamin M" (ibuprofen) for most ailments in the active duty population, once they separated or retired, the Veterans were treated with the more potent meds – narcotics. Yet, with new legislation passed, the rug had been all but pulled out from under those Veterans, as the VA providers had practically ceased prescribing any and all narcotics.

In essence, the providers had prescribed very large doses of narcotics to Veterans for *years*, (maybe the thought was that if the

Veterans were *stoned* then they wouldn't care that their providers couldn't figure out what was truly wrong with them) and then after the passing of the new law, instead of **weaning** those Veterans off of their *hefty* dose of narcotics, they (the providers) had just either terminated those prescriptions or cut back the doses significantly.

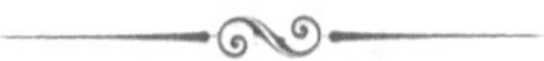

THIS EXAMPLE WAS ANOTHER where a Veteran was prescribed a rather large dose of narcotics, this one had been on hydrocodone for **years**. If I remember correctly, it was something to the effect of 20mg every 6-8 hours daily. Then his provider, without consulting with or *even* informing the Veteran, refilled his medication with only **one quarter** of his normal dose. Let's hear it for the lawmakers! Hooyah! And Hooray for avoidance!!! **Not!!!**

The reasoning why this one Veteran had been taking narcotics was that he was having diffuse and chronic pain (basically all over his body) for years. This little old man was somewhere in his seventies and had told me he had been exposed to Agent Orange during the Vietnam War. The other five members of his squad had all passed away from some form or another of cancer. This gentleman informed us that he had been suffering with this all-over chronic pain for years. Still, he was able to control it with the use of his normal daily dose of narcotics. He stated he did not want to know where he had cancer, he just knew he had it and was going to die, but he was not sure when. He said he didn't care where it was and he didn't want to find out and try to treat it as he was the only one left of his squad, and all the others received treatment and still passed away from the cancer. He told me he didn't need or even want to know where he had cancer because he had no desire to try to fight it. He figured it was too late by the time he came into our clinic. He knew it was a futile struggle trying to fight something he knew would only kill him in the end. He stated he would just like to remain as comfortable as he possible be until he passed.

I contemplated how extremely strong that gentleman was, and I completely agreed with his thought processes. What was the point of doing all sorts of heroic measures, including tests and treatments, only to possibly suffer more during the process of fighting something that would probably be more painful and ultimately have the same outcome?

His Primary Care Provider cut his pain meds down to one quarter the dose that he had been taking for *years,* all in the blink of an eye. Most people may be able to imagine what that would do to someone who had been taking long-term narcotic pain medications, especially an elderly individual. Although it may not kill him, I was sure he'd probably wish he were dead. Might as well just have killed him then! (***Oh. My. God***. That was so not a threat! For any fanatics out there who have absolutely no idea what sarcasm is. In fact, by the time of the writing of this book, this gentleman had probably already passed on, hopefully peacefully.)

Once again, I digress. Our provider did what they could to assist the individual. Unfortunately, even contacting the *Acting* Chief of Staff did nothing to alleviate the Veteran's concerns. It was sad really, considering that the upper *management* would jump through hoops to coddle *a twenty-something Veteran who spent a whopping nine months in the military and somehow was granted 90% disability without even getting out of basic training.* But, they would do absolutely nothing for someone that spent time fighting a war for our country. It was almost as though the more one pushed and complained (bitched and moaned) the more that was done do for them – the squeaky wheel gets the grease and all. Additionally, those older Veterans (for the most part) were relatively passive/compliant and just seemed to go with the flow, mistakably thinking full well that the staff at the VA medical centers were concerned with doing what was in the Veteran's best interest.

That was one of my biggest regrets with leaving, not being there to advocate for my fellow Veterans. But, the VA where I worked was so extremely damaged that it was going to take more than lil 'ole me to try and fix what was broken. That VA needed a total overhaul to fix what was wrong with it. Additionally, when *management* didn't care to do what was in the best interest of the Veterans, that was never going to happen. Needless to say, this was one of the heartbreaking stories that did not have a happy ending. The clinic (and overall the VA) basically failed that Veteran and left him to his own accord to handle his chronic, almost debilitating pain. This meant him being on his own with only a quarter of the dose of medication that he had taken for years. All without so much as a 'thank you for your service, and I hope this pain doesn't kill you' attitude. ***Disgraceful!***

Orange

I had begun to realize that most of the Veterans I encountered and written about thus far were those that I had come across during my time working in triage. That was either because I was triaging *a lot*, or because those Veterans were the most interesting of the bunch. Then again, it was probably since I spent *a lot* of time triaging. Additionally, most of the time was not even discussing what ailed those Veterans, but rather listening to them talk about their time in the service. Honestly, it was hard to tell. Several Veterans I encountered didn't even have a valid complaint. Some just came in because they were lonely and wanted someone to talk to in order to have some human contact, or just a friendly face to make them smile. Unfortunately, they were stuck with me. ☺

AT ANY RATE, LATE ONE morning, I had the extreme pleasure, and sadness, of talking with yet another Vietnam Veteran who presented to triage, sat down and we just started talking. Frankly, to this day, I do not even remember why he had come into the clinic to be seen, or if he even wanted to be seen. But I must've spent a good thirty minutes with him in triage as he spoke of the horrors of Agent Orange. (One thing I will genuinely miss about working at the VA was the chance to listen to the stories Veterans occasionally tell. Those stories are as much for them as they are for the listener. They are not stories one will ever hear from someone who has never been in the military. If ever given the chance to sit and talk with a war Veteran, take heed. It is not something experienced by just anyone.)

MANY PEOPLE HAVE HEARD the term, Orange, in relationship to the Vietnam War. Yet, for anyone who doesn't know what Agent Orange is, you're not alone. I, myself, had to research it, but nothing could describe it with any justice more than a Veteran who experienced what it had done first-hand. The horrors of Agent Orange can be researched all day long, and yet until speaking with someone who lived through the horridness of it will never seem real. Allowing a Veteran who lived through the misery, a chance to relay their experience out loud will not only offer them the cathartic release, it will provide a significant insight into what those Veterans suffered.

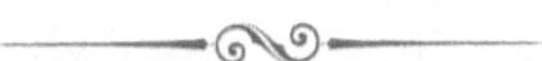

THAT *young* man told me that his squad was on a hill patrolling in Vietnam for thirty days. Every day they would march up and down that hill, watching the area. Then, one night his squad had all gone to sleep, on that very hill. During the time they slept was when the Agent Orange was dropped. To illustrate, from what I could ascertain, Agent Orange was a herbicide on crack. It would kill **everything** in its wake, somehow sparing the troops sleeping on the hill. The very next morning when the squad awoke and started their daily patrol of the hill, the Veteran noted that absolutely **nothing** was left in the area along which they were making their rounds.

"All of the trees were gone. No animals were around. Not even one blade of grass was left on the ground," he stated with a faraway look in his eyes, bringing tears to my eyes.

The way he described not being able to see one single blade of grass that survived the explosion/dusting/drop, or whatever it could be called, on an entire hill, was definitely concerning. It was also somewhat helpful in understanding some of the medical issues those Veterans exposed to Agent Orange experienced, or even still experience.

Reflecting back to that day, I believe, he (as many others exposed to Agent Orange) complained of having a bit of breathing issues. Of course it was not an emergent issue with him. (Duh, if it had been, I would not have kept him in the triage room for so long talking. Nor could I think that he would've been able to carry on a conversation for very long). We continued to talk some more, for a time, and that was when I had my eyes opened even wider than if I had read the facts for myself.

He would stop for brief moments to catch his breath, and during those times I swore I could've seen some tears forming in his eyes. I asked him if he was okay, and he would respond, "This, right here, is better than any medicine they (meaning the VA) can give me. The ability to be able to talk to someone about what we went through, helps more than you know."

I had no idea how to respond to that, nor could I, as I was tearing up myself. All I could do was hold his hand until he felt as though he was done. When he had finished his story, he thanked me and got up to walk out. I felt the need to ask, "Sir, do you need us to do anything for you today?"

"No ma'am. You've done more than you know just listening to my old soul talk."

After he left, I quietly teared up a bit for all the lost souls that couldn't be saved.

My suggestion to whomever, if *ever* given the chance to talk with a Veteran from the Vietnam Era, or if even luckier to meet and have the opportunity to talk to someone from World War II, just sit, and listen. Those Veterans have some of the most amazing, and sometimes heart breaking, stories to tell; all one needs to do is listen. Oftentimes that is all they want. Think of all the things that could be learned from an experience such as that. It is truly nothing one could ever learn from a history book, and it will enrich one's life more than anyone could ever know.

You Can't Help Me!

As in any Emergency Room I've ever worked in (albeit this was just a clinic) we were required to orient to the floor before being able, or required, to conduct triage. (That was most likely to allow one to get the feel of how things were run in each different facility.) To reiterate, I did say this place was not like most, as things were done differently than any other place I'd worked, although it **was** more or less a walk-in clinic, versus an Emergency Room. I could usually triage with my eyes closed; however, when it came to documenting the information, I wanted to know where everything needed to be documented correctly in the chart. I would have liked a few weeks to have been able to navigate the computer charting system before I was tossed into triage. It was a pain in the ass to have to *hunt and peck* (or – as Bertha stated – I so *inappropriately fumbled* my way) through a new charting system while trying to sort amongst the patients and determine each complaint and acuity (severity) in addition to getting everyone seen in a timely manner.

Unfortunately, I was not afforded the luxury of learning the computer system, let alone given any kind of orientation on the system, prior to being required to triage. Since we were consistently short-staffed (yes, that's right, I said it yet again, we were regularly ***short-staffed*** which was par for the course during the entire time of my employ), I ended up in triage within the first few weeks I worked in the clinic. The primary reason was mainly because our *fearless leader* (more sarcasm) allowed one of the RNs to go on vacation, leaving myself and one LVN, who was not trained to triage as it was not in the scope of practice for LVNs. Oh well, as has been said before, (in the military that is, certainly *not* the VA) **adapt and overcome,** or better yet **Semper Gumby**.

Back in triage. One of my very first patients was a male Veteran. To this day I still have no freaking clue as to why he needed to be seen. Apparently, (as I learned **after the fact**) he had a considerable issue with females in general. Obviously, that was a personal issue, of which, who knows if he ever got over it. I digress. I escorted the gentleman into the triage room and just as I sat down at the computer I began by asking, "What brings you into the clinic today?" Indicated for him to sit down opposite me.

Followed by, "How can we best assist you today?"

His butt barely hit the seat when he jumped back up and burst out with, "You can't help me! What makes you think you can help me?"

Taken aback and almost rendered speechless from shock at his completely unprovoked outburst,... almost, I then asked calmly, "Sir, if you'd just tell me why you are here today, I'll see what we can do to assist you."

"You're a new nurse, aren't you?" Entirely ignoring my request for his complaint.

I thought to myself, *Do I freaking look **new**???* I mean, I certainly didn't look like a young nurse fresh out of nursing school. Taking a slow calming breath, I stated, "No, I've been a nurse for many years. However, yes, I am new here at the VA."

"You can't help me!" He repeated, all but shouting that time.

The thought repeating in my head was, *Well okay then. What the Fuck are you doing here? There's the door, don't let it hit you in the ass on the way out.* However, I could not voice those thoughts out loud, so I resorted to calmly stating, "Well, why don't you let me be the judge of that? Tell me what brings you into the clinic today."

By that time, he was getting visibly agitated, akin to a caged tiger, and more verbally aggressive. He stood up, pointed his finger at me and shouted obscenities and overall basically inappropriate statements that were not relevant to any type of medical issue, unless he was having a psychotic break, which (I found out later) was not the case. From my vantage point by the wall, as he faced me (and the wall behind me) I had a perfect view of the door and the hallway beyond. The hallway had filled up with people probably wondering what in the world all the yelling and commotion was about.

I then proceeded to walk around behind the Veteran, to the door, closing it to give him a little privacy. (The hallway filling up went back to many of the staff at the VA not having jobs and therefore not having much to do during the day. So, why not violate HIPAA and patient privacy and add a little more information for their afternoon gossip sessions). The Veteran then became much louder to the point that one of the cops poked his head into the triage room. By that time, I was trying very hard not to laugh or appear as though I was not being completely professional and concerned about the Veteran's needs. After all, he was the one that came to us for help but would not allow us to assist him. The cop that poked his head in proceeded to walk further into the room asking as he went, "Is everything okay in here?"

"Yep. Everything's just fine," I stated rather calmly.

"No, everything is not fine!" the Veteran practically yelled. "This lady cannot help me and I need help!"

"What do you need her to do?" questioned the cop.

"It doesn't matter, she can't help me."

"Let's come out in the hallway and talk. Let me see if we can't figure out what you need," the cop stated to him, apparently placating the Veteran enough to leave the triage room.

As the Veteran walked down the hallway, away from the clinic, with the cop, one of the nurses I worked with came in and asked me, "Are you okay?"

"Me. I'm fine," I stated, starting to chuckle. Meanwhile closing the door behind us in order to maintain some semblance of professionalism. "***Oh, my God***, it was so hard not to laugh while he was in here. I honestly have no idea why he is even here. He would not give me one hint as to what he wanted."

By that time, we were both in tears from laughing so hard.

"Well, I am glad you are okay. We heard the yelling all the way in the back and were wondering what was going on. Of course we had to come and find out what all the commotion was about."

"Yeah, that's happened to me before. But wow, he was like one of my very first patients and now we're are all backed up because he took up so much of my time and for what? Now I am behind." (And *still* freaking learning the computer charting. Ugh!)

How does someone deal with that? A patient being confrontational and, in a sense, verbally attacking, not wanting to voice what they needed. Yet, that same person also becoming completely miffed that no one could help them. Truly, how does that work? The only thing I could do was joke about it because it was entirely laughable. Someone came into my place of work, requested assistance, and then verbally attacked me ***and then*** didn't even tell me the reason why. Ludicrous, I tell you! I do believe that the cops escorted the Veteran from the facility that day. I don't recall having anymore interactions with him during the rest of my time employed at the VA.

I Need Oxy

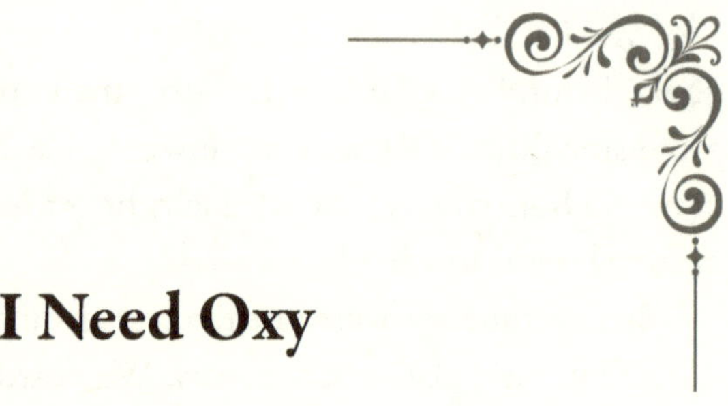

Late one afternoon, about an hour before closing time, a Veteran, I'll call him Jerry, presented to the check-in clerk as most all have done in the past, and was the procedure to be seen. I received a *heads up* from the clerk that Jerry was in the waiting room, pacing and demanding refills of his narcotic pain medications. As helpful as most of our admin clerks were, this one pulled up the Veteran's medication list to prepare us for his visit. Apparently, Jerry had been down at the pharmacy requesting, no, rather demanding, a refill. As was par for the course, however wrong it was, the pharmacy would send the Veterans to our clinic, rather than the Veteran's primary care provider, to be taken care of, knowing full well that we were not allowed to refill any narcotics for Veterans on chronic pain management. But, our clinic was the *catch-all* for the rest of the facility, including the ancillary services: pharmacy, lab, and radiology as well as the primary care clinics—and particularly Mental Health. God forbid any of the other clinics saw their own Veterans without an appointment, **especially** when it was nearing the end of the day.

Getting back to Jerry, as it turned out, he had been prescribed over three-hundred tablets of a large dose of Oxycodone **each** month, for I don't know how long.

AS A SIDE NOTE, THE VA had been prescribing Veterans buttloads of narcotics for years and then in the months that I started working there, the providers at the VA were *encouraged* by the federal government to wean the Veterans off all narcotics. The Federal government must've thought it would be a hoot to see those same Veterans withdrawal because the government put more stringent restrictions on the prescribing of narcotics. In addition, they made it illegal (or whatever) for Veterans to obtain narcotics from anyone other than their primary care provider, possibly for continuity of care, who more or less became the *gatekeeper* of the narcotics. This made it somewhat difficult, in a way, for Veterans to obtain their routine pain meds.

Sadly, some Veterans were just plain indolent and instead of going through the proper channels, would do what a lot had done, and used a walk-in clinic as a convenience instead. That thought process must've been that we would just cut corners and refill any and all medications, just to appease those Veterans. That was not the case. In fact, numerous times I actually had to explain to certain Veterans that I, as a Veteran myself, fell under the same rules. When I needed a refill of my medication I have to go through my primary care clinic, also. Unfortunately, that didn't usually sink in, although once in a while it did.

NONETHELESS, JERRY ended up having wrist surgery (of all things) recently. Wait..., that *recently* had been ***three weeks*** prior to his arrival . Then, after his surgery he was prescribed an additional ninety tablets of Oxycodone to help alleviate the post-surgical pain. He normally took twelve tablets a day, or rather over one-hundred milligrams a day, and yes, amazingly he was still walking ***and*** driving. He could have very well been over-medicating himself with his usual daily dose as well as the additional meds he had been given. I kindly (as possible), which I might mention was quite difficult in between his bouts of yelling and arguing with me, informed him that we would not be able to refill his narcotics. I tried to apologize for the pharmacy screw-up by sending him to us in the first place.

Jerry did not want to hear any of it unless we stated, *Sure, we'll refill your Oxycodone, and we'll give you as much as you want.* That seemed to be all he wanted to hear, and until we actually said those words, he seemed to not listen to reason. Considering we would not be able to accommodate him, he then literally would not shut up and allow anyone to get a word in edgewise. We attempted to inform him of the procedures for competent medical care, as well as the VA's policy. It got to the point that we ended up calling the VA cops on him. Although, they might've even heard the commotion down the hall from their office and just came to check it out. Frankly, I don't even remember, nor was it relevant. Either way, the fact that the cops showed up became a huge predicament because by that time Jerry thought we were all *ganging up* on him. WTFE (What the Fuck Ever)!

As soon as the cops arrived, Jerry all but yelled, "So, what? Are you going to arrest me now?"

"Sir, we are not here to arrest you, but you do need to calm down and let these people take care of you. Your agitation is interrupting the care of the rest of the Veterans here that are also in need of medical care," calmly stated the Lieutenant.

"I just need my Oxy refilled, that's all I need. Can't they do their job and help me get this refilled."

Luckily, by that time, the clinic had just about emptied out and Jerry was our last patient of the evening. I approached him at the nurse's station (as he was extremely agitated and would not remain in the room we had assigned him) on his level, Veteran to Veteran. Unfortunately, that approach (nor any other) worked with Jerry.

"Sir, what do you need the narcotics for?" I asked, probably playing with fire. And to keep poking the bear, I had to add, "What else have you tried for the pain?"

Extremely physically, as well as verbally, agitated he ripped off his wrist brace and almost threw it at me, yelling, "I **HAD WRIST SURGERY!**"

Attempting to remain as calm as possible (as well as trying desperately not to laugh out loud) I stated, "I don't need to see your surgical scar. I just asked what you needed the pain medicine for."

"I told you, I had surgery," he practically screamed.

"How long ago was the surgery?"

"Three weeks!"

"Let me get this straight," I began quizzically, "you had surgery on your *wrist, three weeks ago* and you are still needing additional pain medication? More than your normal twelve tablets a day?"

"Yeah! That's what I've been trying to tell you folks!" Jerry continued, yelling.

"Three weeks ago? (pause) For wrist surgery?" I was baffled. "Sir, I had major open abdominal surgery twice and each time I was not on narcotics for longer than a week or two. So, you've got two choices here. One, you can walk out of here and go home and talk with your primary care provider in the morning (as it was way past clinic hours by that time) or Two, you can get detox treatment to get you off of the narcotics once and for all. Your choice."

"You're not going to give me any more Oxy?"

"That's right. For starters, we are not allowed to refill narcotics as it is your primary care provider's decision, not our job. Also, you have not been taking them as prescribed either. **No. More. Oxy**. However, you can contact your primary care provider in the morning and take this up with them and see if they will refill your Oxy."

"But, I'm in **PAIN!**" He all literally whined.

Again, feeling as though I was banging my head against a wall, I asked, "What else have you tried for the pain?" That of course fell on deaf ears.

By that time, it was no different that talking to a drunken college student while being completely sober, or trying to reason with a toddler having a tantrum. Similar to banging ones head against a wall repeatedly, to the point of getting a headache. I would soon be needing the Oxy myself. I just looked at him, hoping the lightbulb over his head would suddenly flash on and he'd come to the realization that we were not going to appease him by refilling his medication. The whole time Dr. Fitzgerald was sitting at the computer, facing the windows, typing up charts. I caught her looking at the reflection (because by that time it was dark outside and the window was functioning as a mirror) of the scene unfolding behind her at the nurse's station, and smirking.

At one point, a VA cop was positioned behind the Veteran. I was in front of him, attempting to placate him, (and hoping at the same time that he didn't try to take a swing at me), and another cop was positioned next to me. It finally came down to me walking away, hands up shaking my head and telling him that we would not do anything for him unless he wanted to go into a drug treatment program (which he refused) or he could leave on his own accord and take his medications as prescribed and get his monthly refill when the time came for it to be refilled. I needed a break by that time. I was too old to deal with the damn drama and especially a hyped-up Veteran that would not listen to reason, and possibly even stoned out of his gourd.

I walked out of the clinic and went to the check-in clerk's desk to decompress. The next thing I knew, Jerry was walking out of the clinic, followed closely (however not being officially escorted) by the cops. Down the long hallway to the entrance to the clinic they went. Good riddance! It really was difficult to help some people, especially those that didn't want to help themselves.

It's All About Me!

In the previous chapter, the VA Medical Center was described as being notorious for *not* doing what was in the best interest of the Veterans, unless of course that Veteran just so happened to cause a ruckus. An incident occurred shortly before my resignation when Dr. Dumassé showed up to the clinic informing our staff that there would be a Veteran, Cameron, coming in from one of the CBOCs (Community Based Outpatient Clinics) over an hour away, who would basically be jumping the line (rushed to the front of the line). The reasoning was Cameron **demanded** to be evaluated and treated for a simple issue that could very well have been handled at his primary clinic level, and should have been. But once again, *management* was notorious for **not** doing what was right. We all knew by that time that they (*management*) did what was in their best interest and **not** what was in the best interest of all Veterans.

All Cameron needed was an evaluation for a **chronic** orthopedic injury which he attained **prior** to his even enlisting in the military. Nevertheless, the military *did* accept him and therefore were required to take responsibility for the injury. (Although, it was probably **not** disclosed on the part of the Veteran during his initial evaluation into the military, at MEPS – Military Entrance Processing Station). The reason I mention this was because Cameron stayed in the military for less than a year. That didn't even give him enough time to get out of his initial training, let alone be deployed, prior to his separation from the military. Furthermore, because of his somewhat *fraudulent* (aka lies by omission) enlistment he made a significant fuss and somehow, allegedly, ended up having a 70-90% disability rating. Being the young, twenty-something, man that he was, I knew his training could not have been nearly as stringent as it was thirty-plus years ago. It was certainly doubtful that he was injured while in basic training. With the new *kinder-gentler* military and all the *training time out* and *stress cards* those days, his injuries were almost guaranteed to **not** have been acquired during his time in the military. Had he been in long enough to actually deploy once, I may have cut him some slack, but as it was, he was just a wimp.

As Dr. Dumassé continued on usual his diatribe, we attempted to inform him (as we were sure he very well already knew) that chronic orthopedic issues were not acute issues and there was absolutely no reason we needed to rush Cameron right back as soon as he arrived at the facility. Why would we *roll out the red carpet* for a *boot camp Vet* when we would never even do that for a World War II, a Vietnam or Korean War, or even an OEF/OIF Vet.

Yet, Doctor Dumassé and his haughty, better than thou – no military training – attitude might as well have said *talk to the hand*. Furthermore, he was not well suited to work with people in general, as he did not seem to be one to actually listen well or be able to take the opinions of others into consideration. Nor was he one to follow the policies and procedures of the facility in which he worked. Moreover, Dr. Dumassé was also not one to completely understand how things **actually** functioned in the clinic, or rather, he most likely **chose** not to follow the policy and procedures of the facility and subsequently our clinic.

Frankly, I was **surprised** that they (*upper management*) did not roll out the red carpet for Cameron themselves, and assign one of us (*peons*) to escort him around the clinic. The way they acted, it seemed as if the CNO (Chief of Naval Operations) himself were to show up at our clinic.

I digress, once again.

FINALLY, AFTER SOME nail-biting time (*Ha! Right!*), Cameron showed up, entire family in tow. His wife and two or three kids, as well as himself, probably wondering where the red carpet was, as well as the person assigned to *kiss his ass*. If it does not seem obvious by this time, I was not happy with the treatment that was bestowed on that individual as we have done far less for the Veterans that have given ***a lot*** more to their country and have not complained one iota about the treatment they received, or did not receive.

Promptly on arrival, Dr. Dumassé ushered the entire family into the one room that had the most privacy, and a door that shut. Thank God for small favors. That way we would not have to listen to his bitching and moaning, and the kiddos screaming. Then, only one provider was allowed to evaluate and *treat* Cameron. What's more, it was not Dr. Fitzgerald, the provider actually assigned to our clinic, as she had other, ***real*** patients that needed more urgent treatment. Dr. Fitzgerald was also quite content with not having to kiss some whiney Veteran's ass.

The person ultimately assigned to treat Cameron was a mid-level provider. When I say *treat* I mean the provider (a Nurse Practitioner) had to do what Dr. Dumassé told them to do. Why Dr. Dumassé just didn't evaluate the Veteran himself was beyond all of us, as he remained in the clinic the entire time Cameron was there. No wait, I do know why... it was because again, Dr. Dumassé thought of all of us as his personal minions, and we were only there to carry out his personal (or otherwise, i.e. professional) orders. If I remember correctly, Dr. Dumassé even escorted the Veteran to radiology for x-rays.

The ***only*** time I have ***ever*** done that was when I was a Corpsman in the Navy and we were doing an ***Admiral's*** physical exam. We were told to escort the Admirals from place to place around the clinic. Funny though, even the Admirals usually told me (or whomever had been escorting them that day) that they had done that procedure every year for many years that they were old enough to walk unescorted, although they appreciated the gesture, they did not need an escort. So, that should enlighten anyone as to how much respect I had for Cameron. Frankly, I was surprised that he didn't stop right in the middle of the clinic and throw a grand temper tantrum. That would've made an awesome viral internet video, though.

LUCKY FOR ME, THE ONLY incident I really had to endure with Cameron was to observe his encounter with one of the cops. That occurred in the hallway right outside of the room where he and his *entourage* were situated. It was painfully obvious that after being in the military for such a short time, he had absolutely no idea how to respect anyone, let alone a superior officer. He was extremely loud and rude to the cop, who was a Veteran himself, and was nothing but respectful to Cameron. (Better the cop than me, because I probably would've dropped his ass for stepping out of line and being extremely disrespectful.) As I overheard the interaction, I caught Cameron stating, "You can call me Sergeant."

In response to his outburst, the cop then as calmly and respectfully as I could **never** have been, told this *sergeant* that he needed to remain in his room, let us do our job, and he'd get taken care of.

What? Sergeant? I thought maybe I had heard wrong the first time. However the cop reiterated Cameron's rank. *How in the hell was he in the military long enough to make rank of Sergeant?* Yes, I thought all of that to myself, in my *inside* voice. Actually, I looked at my co-workers and asked them, as well as the cop after he was finished being somewhat berated by Cameron, "How the hell did he make Sergeant when he was only in the military for less than a year?"

The cop's response was simply, "He's not a Sergeant, he just thinks he is, and I'm willing to feed into his delusion just so long as it gets him out of here faster."

Wow, all the more power to the cop, because I had to keep myself from heading over to the couple during the altercation and jacking the Veteran up myself. He wanted to *pull rank,* **Ha!** I would've gone over to him stating *Sergeant, this here is Lieutenant Matt, and I am Captain T, so if you want to play the rank game, then* **we can play that game,** *and you'll lose! Right now you're going to shut the fuck up and do what you're told by your superiors. That way we can take care of you, as well as the twenty other Veterans you jumped in front of because your whiney ass wanted immediate gratification for an ongoing issue that* **you** *have chosen to ignore for years, and you don't want to go through the proper channels in order to accomplish that treatment. So, if you want us to take care of your whiney-ass* **on-going** *issue, then you'll go back into your room, let us do our job and if you have any further questions or problems, this here is Lieutenant Matt, feel free to ask him.* **Do you understand** *Sergeant?"*

Oh, if only... that would've been so gratifying, not only for myself, but for our entire clinic staff, sans Dr. Dumassé. It was so frustrating when Veterans took advantage of the system, essentially bogging it down for those who really needed the VA for their medical issues. Unfortunately, those were usually the silent ones. Of course, those *silent* ones were typically watching from the side-lines. Especially on that day, as we had a full clinic, and many Veterans present got an eye-full and saw first-hand the unscrupulous politics present at the VA. Come to find out, after all of the time and effort spent kissing Cameron's ass, he left with a bottle of ibuprofen and a crutch for his *bum* knee. A simple cure that he could've very well accomplished at the clinic where all of this started, and saved himself a long drive, and us our sanity.

Soritis

On one of the rare days in our clinic when we had the opportunity to treat a female Veteran (there were more those days, yet, still very few compared to the male variety). In any case, on that day we had the unique opportunity to have not just one, but **two** females come in almost back-to-back. Regrettably, I believe they had both come from the same gene pool. (The story about the second female follows.)

As was typical by this time in my employ, I was working in triage when the female Veteran arrived with a very odd complaint. It was a complaint that I had never heard during my entire career as a nurse. I motioned the female Veteran into triage, and before I had a chance to even sit down and ask her what brought her in to be seen, she piped up with, "I have *soritis*."

I must've given her a look that said I was born that day because not only was I completely speechless, I had no freaking clue what she had said. Truthfully, I had **heard** what she said, but I had never, in my life, heard of a complaint called *soritis*. Maybe I heard her wrong. So, questioning, I asked quizzically, "What brings you in today?"

"*Soritis!*" She exclaimed, louder the second time.

"Excuse me?" I still must have heard her wrong.

"It's *soritis*! Haven't you ever heard of *soritis*?" She asked, with a puzzled look on her face.

Hmmm, that definitely was a new one. I was (quickly) trying to rack my brain to figure out exactly what *soritis* was. I've never actually heard of it, but then again, I was relatively new to the VA system and it could be some elusive disease known only in that community. Still, I was not really sure what *soritis* was, and frankly I was unconvinced that it was actually a real disease. But, I could only imagine. I pressed, knowing I could not search the internet for it in front of her without losing face. "I have to say, I've never heard of that. You're going to have to give me a little more information. What kind of symptoms are you having?" (Meanwhile, I knew that there was no way I could know every freaking miniscule disease out there. However, I thought she might just be mispronouncing psoriasis.)

"I have inflammation and a rash all over my body, and all of my muscles and joints are sore. And my friend, who is a nurse, said it's *soritis*."

Ooh, kay... Trying to remain calm and ***not*** laugh out loud I asked, "Are you sure you don't mean psoriasis?"

"No!" She exclaimed. It's *Soritis*!" By that time she was getting visibly as well as verbally agitated.

"Okay." Nuf said. I proceeded to expedite getting her vital signs and finishing up her triage note. I wanted to get her into the back of the clinic as soon as I could, and far, far away from me. I mean, I'd never heard of *soritis* and for all I knew, it could kill her at any moment (unlikely as that was), or she could crack and injure me at any moment (more likely the latter, after all, we were working with trained killers), or it could be contagious. (Yes, a little more sarcasm.) I truly figured it was just her mispronouncing psoriasis, after hearing her symptoms.

Once she was triaged and placed in a room, I gave report to the doctor.

"Ummm," I began, and hesitated, "this lady has *soritis*. She says she's got inflammation and a rash all over her body and all her muscles and joints are sore."

Dr. Fitzgerald, looked at me like I had grown a second head off my shoulder and asked, "Don't you mean psoriasis?"

"Believe me, I asked, several times. She adamantly insists it's *soritis*. I am going back out to triage and look that one up. However, I could almost guarantee you that it is most likely either psoriasis or a *highly* contagious rash. If I find out anything else useful I'll let you know. In the meantime, you might want to order a psych eval also, just saying. I mean, why should we have all the fun?" *Smirk* Hehehe...

"Get out of here. Get back to work, you" Dr. Fitzgerald stated as she shoo'd me away. I think she was just excited to see this *new and interesting* disease process, the mispronunciation of psoriasis, and not kick my ass for bringing the patient to her for evaluation. I did not want to be around for the theatrics of the evaluation, so I left and went back out to triage. I never did see that patient again, even on her way out of the clinic, which was most likely soon after she was seen by Dr. F. I'd have known if we transferred her out anywhere, so it could not have been a horrific disease. Most likely only psoriasis, like we both had thought. I believed that Dr. Fitzgerald was either shocked or overwhelmed, so much that she didn't even tell me what *soritis* was after examining the patient. Hahaha!

It's Highly Contagious, it's Ah... Ah... Cold

The second female Veteran that came in that very same day was a fortyish Veteran with cold symptoms that had been going on for two or three days. As I walked with her into the triage room I asked what kind of symptoms she was having, not extending her different treatment than any other Veteran.

"Sore throat, runny nose, body aches, sneezing, you know... cold symptoms."

Yeah, I know cold symptoms, and I also normally take something for them.

"How long have you had these symptoms?" I asked.

"Oh, about a week now," she told me.

"What have you taken for your symptoms since this all started?" I didn't ask *if* she'd taken anything because I knew full well that, like most patients that I'd seen in an ER for cold symptoms, she hadn't taken anything.

The look I received would've caused most anyone to laugh their ass off. It was as though I had grown a second head (or maybe a third by that time). Apparently taking something for a cold was a foreign concept to many. Yep, and those people continue to reproduce (or have so in the past, and therefore there were many more out running amuck, among us).

"What would I have taken?" She asked as though self-medicating was a foreign concept. That's why I came here to see you all, so that you'd give me something."

That **must** have been someone who had **never** watched any TV and seen all of the plentiful commercials for cough and cold treatments and remedies.

Hence, I opted for a different approach. "So, let me get this straight, you haven't tried anything over the counter to help alleviate your symptoms? Any cold remedies or other medications?"

"Like what?" She asked again.

Oh my God, really? Sad thing was, she was old enough and I was almost sure that when she was in the military they were still handing out *cold packs* at the pharmacy in order to stop the backlog of patients in the clinics. Those *cold packs* usually consisted of pseudoephedrine, acetaminophen and sore throat lozenges. I kindly informed her of the various different over the counter medications that were available to try, including their brand names.

I tried to enlighten her with what I considered basic knowledge, "There are any number of cold and flu remedies which contain decongestants, such as pseudoephedrine, pain relievers, other decongestants and cough suppressants. There are also a bunch of less expensive, generic over the counter cough and cold remedies that you can try."

"But that costs money," she whined.

And there it was…! I was not really sure ***what*** her point was, maybe that she was cheap? Oh wait, I knew. She's served her four (or maybe even just two) years in the military and now she should get ***all*** of her medicines for *free*!

Knowing then that I would not get anywhere with my line of questioning and information passing, I proceeded with her triage. Triaging included obtaining her vital signs, which were totally and completely normal. And, of course as she was female between the ages of ten and seventy, I needed a date of her last menstrual period.

So, my dumb-ass-self felt the need to ask, "When was your last menstrual period?"

"I don't know, the first week of the month?" She stated, more of a question than a statement.

*Are you asking **me***??? "Okay, so last week?" (It was only the second week of the month.)

"I don't know. The first week of the month," she repeated.

Again, I asked, "So, then last week?" What was more, it was only Tuesday of the second week of the month. Coupled with, it wasn't as though that was an entirely **new** question or concept for the *young* lady. She had to have been dealing with the issue every month or so, for oh, maybe the past twenty-five to thirty years, minus any pregnancies, maybe. No wonder she didn't attempt to relieve her symptoms with any over the counter medications, she couldn't even remember when her last menstrual period was, as it was supposedly only a few days prior. Oooh, maybe it was early onset dementia setting in. She was also probably someone who went to an Emergency Room because of menstrual cramps, or chapped lips.

By this time of my triage questioning, I was completely fed up with having to talk to what I could only describe as a wall (although that might seriously have been more amusing). Decidedly, I put a hold on my triage note and escorted her to a room in the back and figured I'd finish up my note afterwards. Considering she didn't seem entirely sure **what** was going on. I could've made anything up and given her a good, plausible reason for actually being in the clinic. I did have to give her kudos though for **not** going to an *Emergency Room* for her (extremely trivial) cold symptoms.

Once we arrived in the room she then felt the need to pipe up, "Tissues". That was all she said, nothing else.

Okay? I was thinking she's might also have some sort of disease that causes unwanted or inappropriate outbursts. Hehehe... So, I asked, "Excuse me?" I truly wasn't sure I actually heard her correctly, or why she was saying *tissues*.

So then she repeated herself. "Tissues," and it wasn't a question, more of a statement.

Oh my God, **really?** **What did she want???** Okay, I knew **what** they were, and what they were used for, as well as the fact that we did have some. The question was, did **she** have any? Was she asking me for them, or was she (*now*) telling me that she had used tissues (as an over the counter *remedy* of sorts) to help alleviate her symptoms? She was the one with the sneezing and runny nose and maybe surprisingly she has none (meaning no tissues). I was completely flabbergasted, and a little pissed off by that time. What I really wanted to do was shake her and ask, **What do you want?** I capitulated. I supposed she could very well have been asking me for some. So, I asked, "You need some tissues, or you used some at home for your symptoms?"

"That's what I said."

Eh, not really. But, I looked through the cabinets and drawers in the room and found none. I could only assume that she could obviously tell I was looking for something, yet found that very precise time to pipe up yet again, with simply, "Tissues."

Seriously, you're forty-something, **use your words** *lady!* So, without a word to her (because my *words* would **not** have been pleasant), I headed off to the supply room with the intention of grabbing a box of scratchy, hospital-issue tissues. I assumed that was what she was asking for, as she never did say anymore. Yet, before I could step out of the room, she finally finished up what I could only assume was her initial question, "Can I have one?"

Really?!?!?!?! Someone with cold symptoms, not taking any medications to attempt to mitigate their symptoms and then had no fucking tissues with them... What the Hell? Trying, without much success, to control my frustration at the *toddler-like* mentality of our newest patient I muttered rather sarcastically, "I'm looking," not caring at all if she heard me or not.

I found a box in the supply room and brought it back to the room, placed it on the bedside table. With that she actually articulated a simple, "Thank you."

Then, I headed over to Dr. Lynn and said, "She's **all** yours, doc. Good luck. She's got a cold and the mentality of a two-year old. But, that's just my opinion."

As it was wintertime, Dr. Lynn had actually brought in several boxes of soft, lotion-filled tissues. She asked me as I was headed out the door, "Why did you give her the hospital tissues? We have nice soft ones here."

"You'll see." Was all I said. I was done with the *toddler* in the house, by that time.

With that, I headed back out to triage to finish up my note. I could feel Dr. Fitzgerald's gaze burning into my back as I walked away from her. Oh well, so not my problem anymore... BAWHhahahaha.....

Funny, shortly after I returned to triage, the female Veteran I had just triaged was heading back out to the lobby, assumedly to pick up her *free* medicine at the pharmacy.

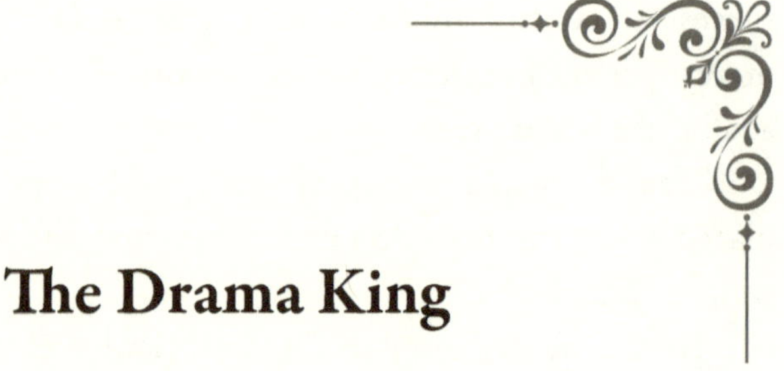

The Drama King

Late one afternoon we had a thirtyish male Veteran limp his way down to our clinic waiting room to wait on a refill of his narcotics that his primary care provider had supposedly ordered for him. (I was not psychic. I found that out after the fact). His primary care provider was in another one of the clinics in the building, but, as it seemed to be the pattern, our clinic was the *catch-all* for anyone who couldn't get what they wanted accomplished from their primary care providers. (That was in-house, as well as in any of the outlying clinics). Or if they couldn't get what they wanted in a timely manner. The Veterans would then come to us in an attempt get things done more expediently.

But, that *gentleman* allegedly was just waiting for the pharmacy to refill his prescription. The reason his story is even included is that he evidently had to wait too long for his medications and apparently got antsy. It seemed as though his primary care provider may **not** have done what they told the Veteran they would do. If people would just do what they said they would do, a.k.a. their jobs*, in a timely manner,* it would've saved a lot of redundancy and frustration on our part, as well as that of the Veterans involved. But, that might interfere with those other staff members' break-times or delay them being able to leave work early.

Nevertheless, the young man had a history of knee, back, and shoulder pain, probably from jumping out of planes and/or helicopters and carrying a hefty-weighted rucksack (backpack), of course, in the military. An occupational hazard. (Not the same individual from a previous story, also with knee pain.)

I was at the admin clerk's desk when he arrived. I watched him limp down the hallway towards the desk and I asked how I could assist him.

"I need my meds!"

Ummm, you just passed the pharmacy. There were two ways in which to approach our clinic, (actually three or four). But, two ways from the primary clinics and one went directly in front of the pharmacy. Surprisingly, that was the route he took.

"What medications are you needing?" I asked, although then regretted even opening my mouth.

"My Hydrocodone. My primary care provider said they ordered them, but that was thirty minutes ago and I am still waiting! Can you help me out?" He shamelessly asked.

"Well, if your primary care provider already ordered a refill, we are not able to piggyback on that and order you anymore. Also, if you are on narcotics for chronic pain management then we wouldn't be able to fill them anyway," I informed him.

He then began arguing that he has been waiting for over a half an hour for his medicine and wanted them now! "Why is it taking so long? Can't you just order some for me and then I'll go pick them up?" He asked.

I began with telling him that if we cancel the order from his primary care provider and reorder the medicine, then he'd be starting over from the get-go with respects to waiting. He evidently did not want to hear that. But, I reiterated **why** we could not order narcotics for patients on long-term pain management therapy. Furthermore, I apprised him, "If you read through the pain contract you signed prior to being able to receive narcotics, as well as having signed yearly, it states specifically that if you are on long-term pain management, which includes narcotics, then you cannot get narcotics from anyone other than your primary care provider. If you do, say go to an Emergency

Room or here in this clinic in attempt to get more narcotics, then you can lose your privileges and your primary care provider will not fill them for you again."

With that explanation, the young man became noticeably agitated and started threatening, no one in particular. However, I was not in the mood to deal with his drama then. Also, What the Hell? He had been waiting a *whopping* thirty minutes to get medications filled. Really?!? It could take upwards of an hour ***or more*** to get a prescription filled or refilled. Local retail pharmacies were notorious for that. I've been in one locally to refill a prescription and the pharmacy clerk would say, 'It'll be twenty minutes.' Then my OCD would kick in and I set my timer for twenty minutes (hoping it'd be quicker). I returned to the pharmacy, only to be told it'll be another twenty minutes. That could go on for hours, but after one time of that, I would request my medicine or refill and then just go home and return the next day, hoping the prescription would at least be filled by then.

I digress. I guess the younger generation was not taught patience in boot camp, or anywhere else. The unwritten military motto was *Hurry up and **wait***. So, instead I told that young man, "Let me see what I can find out for you." Part of my thinking was to get away from him before he tried to ask me to do something else that I wouldn't be able to, or want to, do for him. Before heading off, I asked, "Who's your primary care provider? Which clinic?" After he told me, I headed down to speak to his nurse.

By the time I returned to the admin clerk's desk, not even five minutes later, I noticed he was no longer in our waiting room. Not a minute later I noticed him walking down the parallel hallway from the pharmacy. That time with no discernable limp and in no apparent distress, ***at all***. Apparently, his name showed up on the screen indicating that his medications were ready for pick-up while I was gone. As I observed him walk, I detected no noticeable limp or anything that would indicate that the Drama King was in any pain, like we noticed when he first arrived at the admin clerk's desk. Hmmm... interesting. As soon as he saw me though, his walk suddenly changed. He slowed down and he started noticeably limping once again. Seriously, did he really think I'd buy that crap? I looked directly at him and I knew he noticed my facial expression because he made sure I saw his limp and he held up his baggie of *goodies*, (medications) and said, "They finally got them filled."

"Uh-huh. Good to hear. Guess it pays to wait, huh?" I just couldn't help the sarcasm pouring out.

Ignoring my comment, he limped around the admin clerk's desk and out the back door.

As soon as he walked out the door and around the corner out of eyesight, I darted behind the admin clerk's desk to view the security camera feed of his progress to confirm my suspicions. I was almost convinced I saw him walking without any difficulty or noticeable limp coming from the pharmacy, but I could've been mistaken. After watching him walk/limp out the door, he then start walking completely normal (without any difficulties at all) once he cleared the first set of doors. As we watched on the closest security camera to his location. I pointed it out to the admin clerk, and he said, "What?"

"He's walking just fine. Do you see a limp there?"

"No. He seems to be strutting."

"Exactly! What dramatics." Certainly not the best theatrical display I'd seen over the years. Yet, it was pretty damn convincing if one was not privy to the *before and after* demonstrations of ambulation. Those, unfortunately, were the Veterans that usually made the most *noise* and have the least amount of issues, as well as make a bad name for the rest of us.

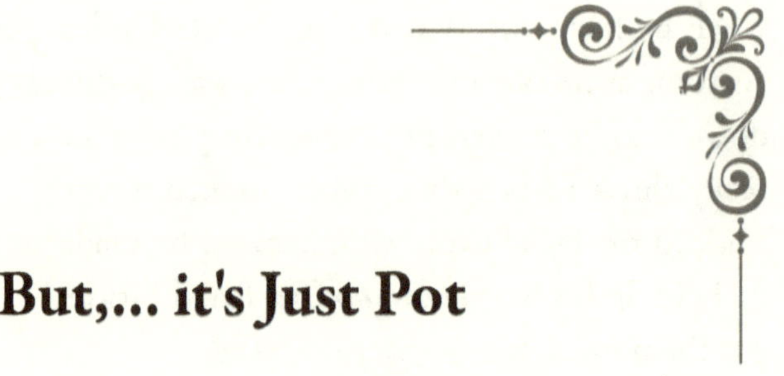

But,... it's Just Pot

Toward the end of clinic hours one day, and during the first hour or so of one Veteran's evening shift working at the VA, he came into the triage room, sat down, and asked if he could have me refill his Hydrocodone. I informed him that we were not allowed to refill narcotics for Veterans that were on long-term pain management. He then asked if I could just check on the status of his refill. He said he had called his primary care provider requesting the refill and the pharmacy said they were unable to refill it for him as of then.

As it was still clinic hours, I contacted his primary care nurse utilizing a text messaging type of system that was available to employees. (I will make it known that I did **not** look through his chart, as his primary care clinic was in the building and I was currently working on another couple of Veterans' charts.) Since his primary care clinic was in the building, and it **was** still clinic hours, I had requested to send the Veteran to his clinic and speak with the nurse. I got a *lovely (yes, that was total sarcasm)* text response from his clinic nurse. The text response I received from his nurse was, "His drug screen was positive, we are not going to refill his medicine."

I pondered to myself... 1. That didn't answer my question as to if I could send the Veteran to see his primary care nurse, and 2. Wasn't it the job of the clinic providers to inform their own Veterans of that kind of information? (Why was it we always seemed to get stuck with their dirty work???)

Since the nurse completely ignored my initial request, I asked again if I could send the Veteran over to speak with her regarding his issue as well as other options for his pain management.

The next text response was not *any* better. "We're busy and the doctor will not refill his Hydrocodone."

And... I'm not busy?!?!? Oh wait, I'd forgotten. That was the one day I was sitting around for hours with my thumb up my ass. (If it isn't obvious by this time, sarcasm has been totally eluded.)

Okay, well then... once again, a patient was *turfed* to our clinic, simply because the other clinics did not want to take care of their own patients, which, frankly, was ***their freaking job!!!***

I then took the time to look through the Veteran's chart on the computer, and pulled up his lab results, specifically the drug screen, and saw that he was positive for Marijuana, Amphetamines, and Cocaine.

"Buddy, you've been self-medicating at home, haven't you?" I asked him.

The look I got said that he had absolutely no idea what I was talking about.

So, I continued, "Your drug screen is positive for several illegal substances."

It was then that I got the most sheepish look imaginable, especially from that particular individual who was normally rude, crude and crass to most anyone and everyone he'd ever met, he didn't discriminate. I'd seen him be crass and verbally abusive to others, however, I have never known him to be that meek and docile, *ever*.

"Dude, you and I both know that *if* you are on narcotics prescribed by the VA, you are not to take narcotic medications from any other providers, nor are you allowed to self-medicate. You signed the agreement before they started you on the narcotics and every year since. I had also signed the same contract and I also have to abide by those very same rules. Your doctor is not going to refill your medications if you are obtaining pain relief from some other source."

Head down and shaking, voice barely audible he asked, "Will they refill it if my drug screen comes back negative?"

"Honestly, I am not sure. That is something you will have to take up with your primary care provider. Do you want us to make an appointment for you to see your primary care nurse to discuss this?"

"No, they won't do anything to help me."

With that, he got up and walked out. I think that might've also been the day when he actually walked off the job without even finishing his shift.

Part III
The Buffoonery Continues

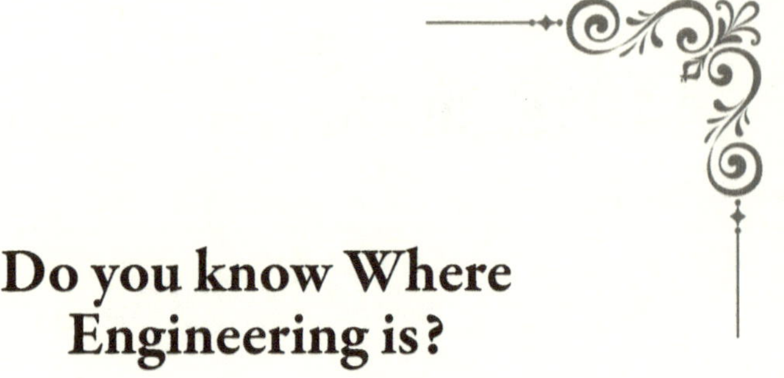

Do you know Where Engineering is?

As I neared the end of my employment with the VA, I resigned my position for numerous reasons. The most notable of which being lack of leadership and accountability. For example, I had left one day at the end of shift, scheduled for surgery the following week, and knowing I would be out a good two months. The day prior, before I left work, Bertha, actually had the *audacity* to say, "You just need to get your surgery done and get fixed so that you can hurry back to work."

I took that to mean she knew I would be gone for two months and that was an inconvenience on her, and the schedule. Additionally, she did not have anyone to replace me for that time, and she was not able to function well enough to fill in, even temporarily, herself. It had absolutely **nothing** to do with any concern she might've had for my well-being. I say this because that was the last time I heard from my *boss* for close to two whole months.

Nearing the time I was due back to work I still had not heard one peep from Bertha. Not one phone call, no text asking how I was doing, or if I needed anything? Nothing! Nada! Zilch! I could have been dead in a ditch and she would not have given two shits, just so long as I reported to work on the day after my leave had expired.

Knowing that and basically not giving a flying fuck, I emailed my resignation and wanted to turn in my keys and badge ASAP so that the VA could hold **nothing** against me.

One day when I wasn't on pain medicine from the surgery, I called the engineering department, knowing that was where I had to turn in my keys, and asked, "I have keys I need to return. Where are you guys located?" (I had never been there, nor did I ever have a reason to go to Engineering, so why would I know where it was?)

"Do you have the keys you need to return?" was the response to my question. *Seriously*!

Taken aback, I wondered if I stuttered or something with my relatively simple question? I'm thought to myself, *Oh My God I just said I had keys to return!* Who *were* those people? I tried to remain calm and not cuss them out for being complete imbeciles. Taking a somewhat calming breath, I restated my question slowly, for the apparent nit-wit on the other end of the phone, "I – just – said – I – have – keys – I – need – to – return, - so – yes, - I – have – them – in – my – possession – and – I – need – to – return – them. Where – are – you – all – located -?" *(That was painful.)*

"Do you know where engineering is?"

Seriously?!?!? That was more painful than if I continuously banged my head against a wall. I wanted to tell that person, *If I knew, would I be calling and asking?* Wherever did they **find** these people?

Taking another not-so-calming breath, I attempted to remain composed. I then informed the person on the other end of the phone, "No, I do not. That's why I am asking you!"

Silence ensued.

Then, more... Silence.

And even more, almost painful, silence. Could that person seriously **not** be able to tell me how to get to their building? The VA campus there was not that freaking huge, there were **maybe ten** buildings total! Unfortunately, I didn't think to ask which building number engineering was located (being out of the military for a few years, I had forgotten about using building numbers. The VA like the military and most government buildings were numbered.) I figured that since the campus was ***not*** that big, it should've be relatively easy to explain to someone where it was and how to get there.

As I continued waiting (somewhat) patiently on the phone, I decided to try my approach another way. I was not wanting to waste any more time on the phone with an obviously incompetent half-wit... I finally asked the person on the phone, "How do *you* get to your office or desk when you walk through the front doors of the VA when you are coming into work?" Head now on the palm of my hands, I was at a total loss if that didn't work. I didn't know how else to find the answer to my question, and subsequently locate engineering.

More silence. I could only imagine what I was dealing with by that time. How do you ask someone where they are located and they have absolutely no clue how to explain it? Seriously, I obviously I had no freaking clue.

So, as even more silence followed, I then tried with, "You don't know how you get to your office, when you come to work in the mornings?" I was flabbergasted by that point, and on the verge of complete frustration. If the person I was supposed to take the keys to did not know how to get to their office, how was I *ever* going to find it?

"Um, just ask the admin clerk when you go into the VA," she finally answered. The admin clerk being the same very admin clerk I worked with on a daily basis. That was also the check in clerk for our clinic and knew me very well. Additionally... they were ***not*** located at the main entrance of that VA Medical Center. I just absolutely *love* dealing with stupid.

I *must* be a glutton for punishment, or in serious need of comic relief. I couldn't hold back any longer, "You can't tell me how you get to your work center when you come into work in the mornings?"

All that person did was repeat the same thing she said previously, "Just ask the admin clerk when you arrive at the VA."

I felt like I was talking to a wall. At that point all I could do was shake my head and laugh my ass off... after all, stupid cannot really be fixed.

Several minutes after I ended the phone call, which could not really be considered a conversation. I drove to the VA and showed up at the check-in desk and asked my buddy how to get to engineering.

"Oh, just go around there (as he pointed down one hallway), out the back door and across the driveway. There's a sign for Engineering on the building across the parking lot. It's like building two or three." Right smack dab behind the main building. Holy crap, that was fucking difficult!!! How challenging was *that* to describe? It was like rocket science after all. No wonder the nitwit could not tell me how she got to her desk/office in the mornings. Ahahaha, apparently extremely grueling for some.

(And the sarcasm continued).

I headed out the way Dave directed, and had no trouble finding the building and location I needed to find in order to drop off my keys. It was a wonder (probably a complete miracle) the person I spoke with on the phone was able to make it to work on a daily basis. Maybe that was why the VA provides five weeks of vacation and two or three weeks of sick leave a year, knowing that they employ people of a certain caliber who were mentally unable to find their own work center day after day. It must've been extremely strenuous, on a daily basis, and therefore certain employees need almost two months of time off a year to recover from the strain of it all.

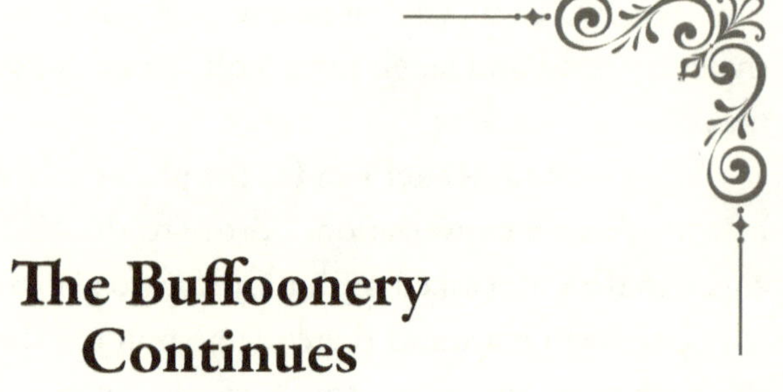

The Buffoonery
Continues

Just when I thought that the VA *circus* has exceeded its limit of rings, it seemed to find a way to squeeze in just one more, allowing the buffoonery to continue.

As I might've previously mentioned, I was also a patient of the VA system. I received a call from my Primary Care Physician one day. I was informed that the referral they submitted previously, for an appointment I've had to have every six months for the past two or three years, was canceled autonomously by a nurse in the Consults department. ***Seriously?!?!?*** First of all, who gave a nurse that much authority to determine which referrals I should or should not have? That was not their job. Their job was to facilitate the appointments, ***not*** cancel the orders.

What did I do? I called Referral Management/Consult Management, (whatever the name was that month) and asked to speak to that particular nurse. Guess what? No answer. So, I left a message. Surprise! No one called me back.

I called again the next day. Still no answer. I left another message and then called the manager of women's health and left two messages (the first one got cut off, so I called back and left my number). It was not going to be my fault if I did not get a return call. Still no response by the next day. (Could it have been that government employees were allotted ***way too much*** time off? Even then, many seemed to be allowed to *play the game* and take more time off without being charged for it, as if they even needed it.) I digress once again.

Fortunately, *someone* from the VA called later the following day.

"Hi, this is Dale from the VA." That was wall he said, by way of a greeting, when I answered the phone.

That was eloquent phone etiquette at its best. It made me wonder when their last secret shopper call might have been. Sarcasm, eye roll,

...

Like most major medical centers or large clinics, that VA was rather large and I had been waiting for responses from a few individual requests submitted by my Primary Care Provider. There was no way of knowing where Dale could've been calling from by his simple greeting. Seriously, I had to wonder where that person was calling from. I figured he was not going to elaborate, so I had to ask (maybe it'd click, although most likely not), "And where are you calling from at the VA?"

For all I knew, and everything I'd been through, it could've been Mental Health calling to check on my mental status. Ha! Who was I kidding? They couldn't do the job they've been tasked to do; did I really think they would *solicit* additional patients?

With a relatively haughty attitude that could've said I should have known who he was as well as where he was calling from said, "I'm calling from Consult Management." I think I even heard an audible Hrmph after his response.

That was a start. "Okay," was all I said as I waited for him to provide me with some additional information.

Complete Silence

After what seemed like at least three to five minutes, Dale finally continued with, "Um, you wanted to know why your referral was canceled, correct?"

"Ah, yeah. Yes. That is correct" I respond.

And then... More silence.

After providing him with a little personal information he requested, Dale then stated, "Well, it states here in the computer that the referral was canceled."

Well, duh! I rolled my eyes to no one but myself.

"*Why*, was it canceled?" I asked pointedly. Sheez.

"Oh, there's no diagnosis in the computer."

Are you freaking kidding me?

Of course, then I had to ask, "So, you're telling me that you all canceled my referral because there was no diagnosis put in? That's just asinine. I've had this same referral every six months for the past two or three years and now all of a sudden you all just cancel it instead of contacting the provider and asking them to put in a simple diagnosis? They're already over-worked, and now they have to redo all the work they had done just because one item was missed and you took it on yourself to just cancel it?"

That's taking care of the Vets for you. Teamwork it was not!

"Well, there was no diagnosis in the referral," Dale reiterated, dumbfoundedly.

"I heard you. Why didn't you all contact the doctor and let them know that they needed to put in a diagnosis instead of just canceling the entire referral? Again, this is something I've had to do every six months and I am expecting an appointment next month. This is completely ridiculous and unsat! All you all had to do was call the provider and ask them to put in a diagnosis. This is a complete waste of my time as well as my primary care provider's time."

"It was canceled in the computer," Dale again repeated, assumingly trying to justify.

Oh My God, seriously? *Someone* had to go into the computer and cancel it, duh! If my provider had not looked in my chart for another issue I had requested then they wouldn't have seen that the referral was canceled.

"So, were you all planning on letting my provider know that the referral was canceled?"

"I'll give the clinic a call today," Dale added, as if that would fix everything.

"They already know that the consult was canceled. They were the ones that alerted me to the issue. What's going on there? I want this fixed now. I have an appointment in a couple of weeks and this needs to be completed." I was about at the end of my rope with that place.

I was not planning on holding my breath that Dale would actually do what he said he would. So, I called my clinic and informed them of the information, and needed diagnosis. Once again, I was forced to have to waste even more of my time to make sure that the VA did what they said they would, and what they should have done in the first place, their freaking job! One of the many things I learned in the military, as well as a nurse: was to document, document, document. If it wasn't documented, then it wasn't done. Additionally, I sent a secure message in to my Primary Care Provider to inform them of where the stupidity lie.

I supposed my Primary Care Provider was also fed up with the buffoonery so much that they ordered any and *all* tests and procedures possible for that particular issue I was having, not that I had any need for everything ordered. I guess they wanted to make sure I wasn't going to have the same issue in the future.

Stupidity truly cannot be cured! Those that fit the description just get hired on by the VA!!!

I thought there was no way that all of this possibly could get any worse, after all that I experienced at this VA. I was *wrong*!!!

It continued...

Finally

After only working in the Veteran's Affairs Health Care System for less than a year and being able to fill up this many pages with personally observed situations, I can only imagine how much has been screwed up over the years, as my time there was a drop in the bucket compared to many that have stayed on for *decades*. I shuddered for all the Veterans that have to be subjected to this lack of care on a daily, or less frequent, basis.

Reflecting on my time there, overall it was not a bad place to work for the sheer enjoyment of being able to work and care for fellow Veterans. Nonetheless, the leadership, as a whole, is in dire need of a clean sweep. It made me question how some of those people could ever be in positions they were. Like several people have told me over the course of my employ, *It's not what you know that gets you your job, but who you blow*. Shockingly well stated, I may add. Where else could taxpayer's dollars be wasted and people still get paid to do schoolwork during working hours without fear of being reprimanded, or worse, fired? Just so long as the right person was getting screwed, then anyone could more or less get away with anything, even the shoddy care of American's Veterans. Looking back, stupidity almost suffocated me there. Had I not left when I did, I might not have been lucky enough to get out alive, or with my sanity intact.

And now... on to enjoying retirement and starting the next chapter of my life.

THE END

Don't miss out!

Visit the website below and you can sign up to receive emails whenever R.S. Christoff publishes a new book. There's no charge and no obligation.

https://books2read.com/r/B-A-IZQO-XWNTB

BOOKS 2 READ

Connecting independent readers to independent writers.

Also by R.S. Christoff

Stories from the ER
Chocolate Chip Cheesecake... with Nuts in the Crust

Standalone
Darker Shades of the VA

About the Author

R.S.Chistoff is a pen name I have used for this (and subsequent books). I served twenty years in the Navy and Air Force. I am a retired military Emergency Nurse and Hospital Corpsman. I have traveled around the world, to include places stateside as well as overseas. As a Hospital Corpsman/EMT I worked in isolated locations around the world. My stories come from these experiences.